THE 'GO-TO PHYSIO BOOK

David O'Sullivan

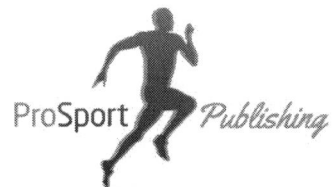

ProSport Publishing

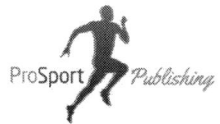

ISBN: 978-1-727-41652-7

A CIP record for this book is available from the British Library

Edited and typeset by Helen Jones

Facebook @TheProSportAcademy
Instagram @ProSportAcademy

Dedication

To everyone that has supported me throughout my journey so far, this is for you.

Georgina, thank you for putting up with me and for the sacrifices you have made and continue to make every single day so I can continue to live my dream. Ava May and Ruby Rae, for being able to take all my problems away instantly with one smile.

Mum and Dad, thanks for all your sacrifices when I was younger to help me get to where I am today, photocopying all the UK physiotherapy university details and driving me to Carlow and beyond for open days…

To all the 'Go-To' Therapist Mentorship clinicians and followers – thank you for trusting in me and giving me the opportunity to help you help people all over the world who have failed traditional approaches.

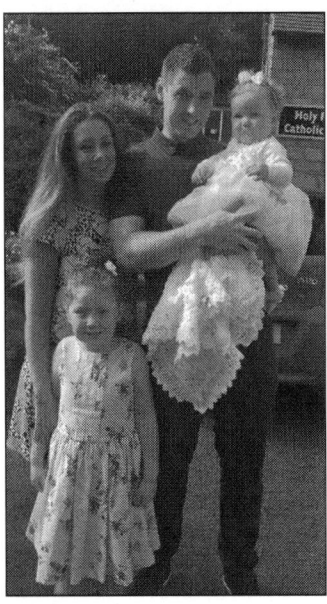

Contents

Before you read the book do this first...

As a thank you for reading this book I would like to give you my *7 Fundamentals To A Successful Discharge* mini course, a video case study for a groin pain patient including videos of the exercises, return-to-play blueprints and worksheets that are mentioned in the book to help you implement this content in the REAL WORLD for maximum success.

Go to: www.thegotophysiobook.com/resources

Here's what you will receive:

- My essential *7 Fundamentals To A Successful Discharge* mini course that will clarify each progression mentioned in the book in even more detail so you can have complete clarity in where to go next with your patient

- Videos of the progressions mentioned in the 'Groin Pain Patient Case Study' mentioned in this book

- Actual real life ACL reconstruction rehab and return-to-play video

- Complete resources from the book, including all the links, return-to-play blueprints and worksheets and even more bonuses that I have not mentioned here.

It's all here:

www.thegotophysiobook.com/resources

You'll need this as you read the book

Go to: www.thegotophysiobook.com/resource now and download your free bonus **Successful Discharge Toolkit** – it contains many of the videos and PDFs of the exercises and progressions I mention in the book.

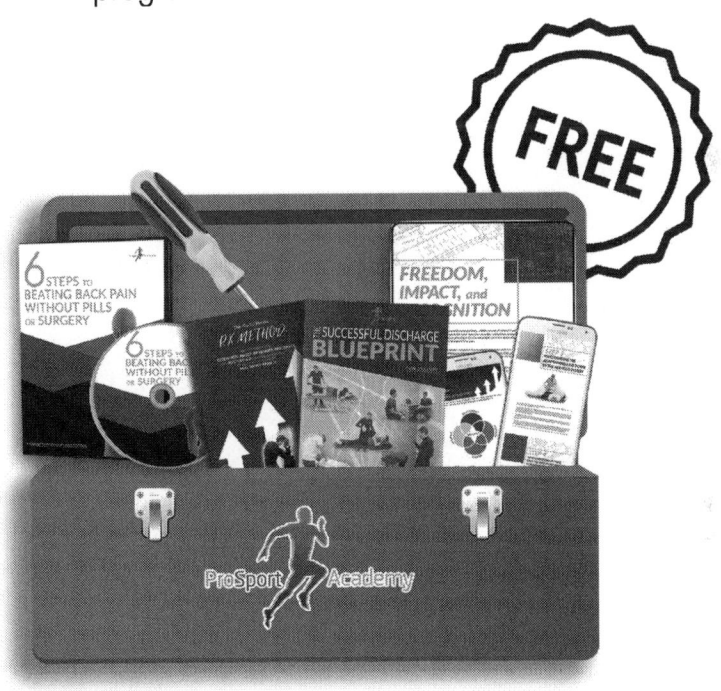

To get the best out of this book download the **Successful Discharge Toolkit** now before you start reading:

www.thegotophysiobook.com/resources

What therapists, players and coaches from all over the world say about Dave O'Sullivan and the Go-To Therapist method

Before joining the Mentorship, I didn't have a clear system in place that I could rely on to get my player from return to play back safe on the pitch.

Joining the Mentorship Dave gave me much better systems in place, a more logical approach where I can work less and even be able to choose what type of patients I want to treat because of my Go-To status in Donegal.

Ronan Brennan, RB Sports Clinic Donegal, Ireland.

Prior to being on the Mentorship I had been following Dave while he was working with the England RL team in the 2017 World Cup and seeing how he got to where he was in his career.

Dave's approach is totally different. He gave me a clear step-by-step approach that I was able to apply straight away on the field with any athlete. I immediately saw the value in what Dave was teaching and made the money back that I had spent on the course in three months.

I was so happy to have a system in place instead of guessing; hands down the best thing I have ever done to move me and my Clinic to the next level.

Anthony Kennedy, North Kerry Sports Injury & Massage Clinic, Kerry, Ireland.

I want to give a thank you to Dave O'Sullivan and his Mentorship as I have just been offered a job with Rotherham United Academy! Before starting this Mentorship I wouldn't have had the knowledge or confidence to even apply for the job! I'm really enjoying it and I can't wait to begin to implement my new knowledge in the job!

Elly Kirk, Rotherham United Academy Football Club, Sheffield, England.

This week my Clinic is at an all-time high with number that I can possibly fit in around my boys and their commitments and this has happened over the last eight months from being on the Mentorship and opening the Clinic. The growth has enabled me to gain confidence in myself I never thought I could achieve. The future can only get brighter; I can't wait!

Katie Evans, Moves Well Soft Tissue Therapy, Cornwall, England.

I want to say thank you once more, because it feels like I've found the missing link. My therapy outcomes have improved greatly. I have gained more clarity where previously I felt lost with my reasoning and I am able to give every patient the exercise they need, so the gap between pain-free in the treating room and going back to specific activity is closing.

Philipp Endl, Austria National Under 21 Football Team Physiotherapist, Austria

Since joining the Mentorship I know exactly what exercises I should be giving out that will eliminate my patient's pain and stop it from coming back. With Dave's business strategy, I am able to just see the types of patients I want to treat and still have a profitable Clinic that's given me the financial freedom I always wanted. Because Dave is all about systems, I have more time to work on maximising my Clinic in a business sense.

Derek Stenson, Midlands Physical Therapy, Ireland.

The Mentorship has massively changed the way I am working; it's given me long-lasting results, and my patients love it! Once they see the results, straight away their skepticism just totally disappears.

My confidence has improved loads in terms of treating my patients, thanks to Dave. Dave has helped me to understand their story; my skills have gone above and beyond. Dave's course is a revelation in so many ways – I can't recommend it enough.

Colin Gordon, Performance Sports Therapy, Edinburgh, Scotland.

Dave really changed my mindset and the way I think about patients. I have learnt so much from Dave in just these few months of being on the Mentorship. He has given me the confidence that ensures my patients buy into pretty much every treatment plan I give. I am now working a lot quicker, smarter and my time management has improved dramatically. I don't have any stress or pressure on myself; I'm so happy. Thanks Dave!

Eoin O'Sullivan, Private Physiotherapy Practice, Cork, Ireland.

The Mentorship is fantastic! Dave is a genius; his approach is completely different to any other course I have been on. I just couldn't believe how little time I needed to be able to pick the content up and apply it with my patients. He tells you the information in an honest way, without any time being wasted.

Peter Connell, Halifax Rugby League Soft Tissue Therapist, England.

Dave welcomed me with open arms to his Physiotherapy Clinic when I was training up. I told him from the start where I wanted to be in my career and he made sure he helped me get there. Working closely with Dave on his Mentorship I was able to develop a real understanding and advanced clinical skills I could apply. I knew Dave would see me through with all of his past work having his own clinic, teaching programme and working with Huddersfield Giants, England Rugby League. I am just so thrilled he stuck by me. Cheers DOS!

Will Franklin, Leeds United Football Academy Physiotherapist, England.

I was wanting to further my training after coming home and was researching sports physio masters around Christmas but none were really fitting into what I was looking for. I then came across an ad I saw of Dave working with England Rugby League. After I spoke to Dave and found out all about the Mentorship I decided to go with that because of the practical component and it was all knowledge I could apply clinically, straight away. Also a big draw for me was the online community and facebook group for support!

Maria Keane, Private Physiotherapy Practice, Galway, Ireland

I really loved how Dave had a structured programme. He followed a complete step-by-step approach that attracted me and I knew from the first instance it would be something myself and my Clinic would benefit from. It has really helped my confidence with my step-by-step guide and the exercises I give to my patients. I couldn't believe how simple it was to follow yet it was very effective so it was a massive win-win for me!

Yvonne Galvin, GPS Physiotherapy, Co Offaly, Ireland.

Dave is a genius! Since the beginning of 2017, when I had the pleasure of learning from him and being able to meet him in person on his workshops, I could instantly see the passion he has for Physical Therapy and sharing his successful systems with others. No matter where you are at, I can guarantee you will learn something from Dave. I'm never stuck for information and can treat any issue that walks through the door.

Fiona Mernagh, Therapy For Optimal Performance, Dublin, Ireland.

I'm so thankful to Dave; I now go home not being tired from work. It's effortless – so simple. I go to the gym 4–5 times a week. I never thought I would be able to do that. In my first few years of being a therapist, I would just go home – straight to bed. I'm only three months into the Mentorship but I'm absolutely loving it. Dave has been fantastic; he is helping me so much and the amount of time and freedom I have now is giving me such a great quality of life. Every aspect of my life has improved.

Daniel Redmond, Physical Therapy Dublin, Liverpool, England

Dave has given me so much more direction with what I am doing, and really to be honest it's made me enjoy my job a whole lot more.

Alex Bloor, Private Practice, Auckland, New Zealand

Dave's content makes complete sense to me and I just think why haven't we been taught this before? When you actually go through his step-by-step process, and what he has been teaching, it benefits you so much.

Louise Holland, Private Practice, Melbourne, Australia.

The main thing for me was that I could go back and re-watch the videos any time I needed help. Also you can ask any question in the private Facebook page, even with tricky cases and get help from others on the Mentorship. If you want to try a different approach that will get you great results then The ProSport Academy Mentorship is definitely for you.

Melvin Thancanamootoo, Physiotherapist, Melbourne.

The Mentorship has really helped me in recognising and better assessing the connection of hand/wrist to shoulder issues. I was neglecting this way too much in my assessments but with the weekly content in the Mentorship it has really helped me get the results and achieve them much faster.

Seamus Garvey, Physiotherapist, Wisconsin, USA

I saw how quickly Dave climbed the Physio ladder and became the England RL Head Physio and I wanted to follow suit. The Mentorship simplified my work in regards to returning to play so I actually have confidence now in returning my players back to that professional level. When I got really quick results and could keep my players at the level I wanted them to be at, they all started raving about me and how I work. I have a systematic approach to my players now and that translates through the rehab, treatment and getting them back onto the sporting field. I feel like I really am reaching my goal – moving up the elite Sports Physio ladder.

Aaron Turnbull, Sports Physiotherapist, Queensland, Australia

To be honest, Dave and ProSport Academy Mentorship changed my life and boosted my confidence as a Massage Therapist. I feel I am more guided and get more results with my clients/patient.

Menson Lauron, Sports Massage Therapist, Philippines

I had the pleasure of working alongside Dave at Munster Rugby where he was the Senior Team's Physiotherapist. He stands out as one of the best practitioners I've worked with, due to his innovational techniques, knowledge of strength and conditioning principles, and expertise in the treatment and rehab of players.

Aled Walters, Head of Strength and Conditioning, South Africa Rugby

Dave's knowledge of how the body works is second to none. He has a real passion for what he does and always got me back from injury weeks earlier than expected. His combination of rehabilitation exercises, knowledge of strength and conditioning field and his hands-on treatment makes him one of the best clinicians I know. I would highly recommend working with Dave.

Paul O'Connell, Munster, Ireland and British and Irish Lions.

INTRODUCTION

Messing up with Munster Rugby

We left the surgeon's office at about 4pm and headed for the car in an awkward silence. To be fair, the player was upbeat and I could sense almost his relief and a weight lifted from his body.

The drive back to Limerick was also a strange one knowing this would be hitting the national headlines shortly and, essentially, this 'wouldn't' be my player anymore.

Probably, deep down, I was relieved too as I had explored every single avenue I knew (at the time) to try and help him.

But this was one of the few cases I saw on a day-to-day basis where pain truly did mean damage.

And his 'headspace' was right but it could not overpower the signals that were coming from below telling him that the load was exceeding the tissues/ joints capacity to tolerate load for running and change of direction.

To cut a long story short, one of my childhood heroes had retired and I wasn't able to help him.

That hurt my pride and ego a lot, in all honesty, even though I had just joined the team halfway through his rehab plan.

It proved a reality check for me where I certainly thought I was 'close' to being where I wanted to be as a Go-To Therapist who could help people where traditional approaches had failed.

I prided myself on being a very hands-on therapist…

…who would treat 'everything' and leave no stone unturned…

…where players or patients would feel great jumping off the bed but the pain experience or symptoms would return minutes, hours or even a day or so later.

In that year, I had two players retire on 'my watch' and I took that very personally. For one player, pain did mean damage and the load placed on the joint was just too much now for that player to be able to do the one thing he loved doing, while the other player had a 'healthy' body but the constant setbacks proved too much for him.

Here were two players who in reality needed to be managed very differently from the start.

At the time, I brought a very strong hands-on game but a very weak all-round approach to the treatment plan such as managing the person individually. Key components to my treatment plan were missing such as using non-hands-on approaches to reassure the patient, but also having that step-by-step progressive loading plan in place to help show the higher centres of the brain that these body parts can tolerate load once it is applied at the right time and in the right order.

I knew I needed to change my approach and that I would encounter this again if I was too reliant on hands-on treatment to change the symptoms.

So off I went again, on a focused crusade, just like I had done at university, to learn everything I could on what I thought I needed to know more of. I had secured a job in professional sport straight from graduating, but now I needed a more robust system.

This new-found awareness of the problem and the challenges I was having in my day-to-day clinical situations meant that I was reading even older content/resources and chatting to people but was seeing and hearing things differently because I was READY to see and hear it.

This is a very powerful thing and something I see in my private practice business all the time now, whereas in the past I would hear things that would move my business forward but I just did not see the value of that information at the time.

I hope you are ready to hear and see this message and learn from my mistakes.

This method I've now put together is a combination of thousands and thousands of pounds/euros/dollars of courses, Skype calls, reading, travelling in person to meet people and so on.

It is a systematic approach from the minute the person meets you to the minute you discharge them, designed solely to help make a meaningful impact on that patient's life.

And when you don't just get rid of their back pain but have your attention on making a meaningful impact on someone's life, magical things happen for your RESULTS and REPUTATION.

The RETENTION, REFERRALS and REVENUE for your practice all click into place.

You don't need to worry about that patient bad-mouthing your clinic, or dropping off, or not turning up to their appointment because they are highly motivated and want to adhere to your plan and they see you as the authority/guide that is adding real value to their life.

There is a big difference in my opinion between focusing your attention on having a meaningful impact on a patient's life versus just helping this person with their back pain, both for your business success and your clinical success.

It allows you to create a bespoke treatment plan for every patient so they see value in everything they do while also keeping it interesting for you, rather than just giving out the same exercises for the same symptoms for every patient.

But in order for this to happen you need the confidence and clarity of HOW to design your treatment plan and implement it in the real world.

Having that confidence and clarity is also an INVALUABLE skill to have when working in sport as it now allows you to make logical decisions about when that athlete will be ready to return to training or games. This clarity means you know exactly what he/she needs to do to be ready, how many sessions/days/progressions away from this they are now and how quickly you can progress.

This is the reason I enjoyed a relatively stress-free Rugby League World Cup final week in Brisbane in 2017 with England Rugby League.

I had to make two massive calls and I knew deep down that one player would make it and the other wouldn't based on where they were clinically and what we needed to expose them to, to be sure they would be ready.

As the guy who didn't make it went through the step-by-step progressions, and was exposed to situations and load tolerance, he could tell for himself that he wasn't ready. All you will receive is a 'warning sign' usually and the athlete will know themselves that this is the right decision.

In this book it is my intention to share this method with you and help you gain the confidence and clarity that I wish I had back in my dream job in 2012.

All I ask is you keep an open mind and have an awareness of being 'ready' to receive certain information that may initially cause a negative feeling of insecurity within you.

My goal is to help you become the Go-To Therapist in professional sport or private practice that can help make a meaningful impact on people all over the world who have failed traditional approaches.

CHAPTER 1

Why most failed patient treatment plans didn't work with 'traditional approaches'

The 'traditional approach' I was certainly taught in university was to look at the site of pain, perform some mobilisations if appropriate and then load the area, usually with eccentrics.

Now this approach will no doubt get some good results but for the majority of cases I see now that have failed approaches, we need to be thinking 'higher level' and asking some 'higher level critical questions'.
The biggest questions we need to ask ourselves (for non-traumatic injuries) are '**WHY** did this pain experience develop?' and '**WHY** at this tissue?'

For example, why is the Achilles tendon overloaded in one person and the patellar tendon overloaded in another when there is a spike in load or activity?

OR another way to ask this question is '**WHAT** is not contributing to the load sharing or not doing its job well enough?'

The next higher level thinking question is then '**WHY** are these tissues/ joints not doing their job efficiently?'

So, for instance, a patient who came to me last month had had 12 sessions with another therapist down the road for knee pain. He didn't respond to eccentrics, glute work and knee joint loading.

We found through his injury history a previous hamstring injury and the assessment showed that his hamstring was not doing a great job in co-contracting at the knee very well. We had to help the hamstring co-contract which then deloaded the quad instantly and let it worry about doing its job. It also helped the glute max be in a better length-tension relationship by avoiding that 'knee snap back' that you see so often in the clinic.

This is just one example that comes to mind. To give better context, later I'll share other stories of patients who had failed traditional approaches.

Another reason for not getting successful results I see is using the same exercises for every patient who has knee pain or back pain or shoulder pain, for example.

It seems with the availability of so much information and 'exercises' out there on social media these days, the art of assessing and clinically reasoning is slowly dying.

The exercise should serve a purpose to allow the patient to tolerate load through tissues that may have a 'perceived threat' still present, before progressing to the next level of graded exposure (more on this later) and not simply be just thrown at the patient, hoping for the best.

If anything, that approach will actually frustrate you more as some patients will respond while others will not and you will find yourself then losing confidence in yourself and maybe even the exercise.

The exercise was not the problem; it was just that the exercise didn't solve the problem specific to this patient's story.

Another reason for failed results for patients who have come to me in the past is that previous therapists have relied too much on hands-on treatment and have not understood how to truly progress that patient, especially in the higher level rehab and loading.

I've seen this time and time again with patients that come to me after being around the houses and I've seen it personally during my time at Leeds Rhinos and Munster Rugby. A hands-on treatment approach will only get you so far in 'changing the pain experience' but as I like to say:

'Getting rid of pain is easy; keeping pain away is the true art.'

The true ART with patients who have had the pain experience for quite some time is to give them the right stimulus at the right time in the progressive rehab plan.

The final big mistake I see is presuming that an area needs strengthening, and putting a patient through a strengthening programme when it is not actually a strength issue that is the problem.

I have worked with some athletes over the years who were very strong but were still in pain. This whole 'let's just get them strong' mentality just doesn't sit well with me; I think there's a lot more to it than that.

We will discuss this in more detail throughout the book but after ten years of working in professional sport, I believe it is more about coordination than strength.

In this book, I'll share with you how I now look at the person in front of me, make sense of the symptoms and have the clarity to progress the patient through a step-by-step movement plan to tolerate the loads they need to be able to tolerate, to add real value to their life.

Why this is important to sort now

It is important to change your approach to patients now because otherwise you can find yourself just going through the motions and losing interest in the job.

Louise, a good friend of mine, reached out to me and enquired about coming on my mentorship because she had lost the love for her job as a physiotherapist in Australia. Essentially, she was just going through the motions and giving the same exercises day in and day out.

Now her passion for the profession has been reignited. She gets clues from the patient and makes sense of the objective assessment problem solving, using the same method I'll show you in this book. She then creates a bespoke treatment plan for every patient that gets great consistent results, while working with highly motivated and grateful patients.

Continuing down the traditional route without asking some higher level questions can give you a false security of some wins but a lack of consistent results.

We can almost believe we are better than we really are and can make excuses for why patients aren't coming back to us. We can settle for the type of patients who say 'I'll see how it goes and get in touch if I need you again; thanks for everything.'

As your reputation starts to grow and people start to travel for miles to see you, and as a result you increase your prices, you may notice the pressure increases to be able to get CONSISTENT results.

Complex cases, from my experience, will never fit the 'textbook' so having a common sense step-by-step system from the subjective assessment to the higher loading rehab really is the only way to ensure you get consistent results.

Just looking at the site of the symptoms and doing the 'generic' exercises which in reality they've probably already done with some other therapist won't cut it for these patients and you will almost 'lose them' before you even got going.

There is a smarter way to work that will create a stress-free daily working life and business where people will travel for miles or even other countries to see you. This consistent and repeatable system can get results for you.

Typical journey of a therapist

Most universities instill in students the need to READ as many journals as they can and be really critical of the papers; this would then somehow magically transfer into PRACTICAL, REAL WORLD SKILLS.

The therapist continues this approach on their career journey and then pretty quickly gets a shock at the REALITY of working in the REAL WORLD and so learns a few techniques here and there without any substance as to WHY they are doing this technique or how it fits into the overall plan.

Being brutally honest, from speaking to well over one thousand therapists now on calls, mentoring courses etc., the vast majority have no OVERALL plan and are winging it on a session-to-session basis hoping for the best.

Obviously not all are but, for the vast majority I've spoken to, this is their current reality.

They then invest hundreds of pounds/euros/dollars on hands-on treatment courses or some 'technique' course to try and get some positive results.

And this can further fuel the fire and lead them down the wrong path. This was certainly the case for me. I got some quick short-term wins with patients' symptoms and so I used certain hands-on techniques for EVERY patient with that symptom REGARDLESS of their story or ASSESSMENT findings.

For instance, a therapist spends hundreds of pounds on a dry needling course and the next thing on Monday morning every back pain patient is getting a dry needle in the glute medius and the QL.

WHY is that glute medius or QL (in my opinion you are not even palpating the QL, but that's another story for another day) carrying this protective tone or sensitivity in the first place?

How does that fit with the patient's story? Is this even the true cause in the first place or simply a reaction?

The ART of CLINICAL REASONING is slowly dying in my opinion.

So the next problem the therapist encounters is that the patient is getting some temporary pain relief with these hands-on techniques but the symptoms return again or get worse; they go completely but flare up when the patient goes back training or running, or whatever the higher loading activity may be.

So they then book themselves onto a 'Strength & Conditioning' or 'Movement Course' or 'Rehab Course' that will teach a few movements and exercises.

But again, Monday morning, the therapist falls into the trap of 'oh', now every patient is getting this exercise routine.

How does this exercise solve a problem found in the assessment specific to the patient's story and is this the next logical progression in the treatment plan?

Clinical reasoning is king

Whether you are a hands-on or hands-off therapist, you still need the basic ability to clinically reason a step-by-step progressive treatment plan that complements the findings of the assessment and makes sense of the patient's story which is unique for them, to help them be successful in the real world.

Because, ultimately, all that matters is what happens when the person goes out of your nice, safe treatment room and into the real world.

This lack of clinical reasoning and having that step-by-step progressive approach then shows up in a lack of confidence and clarity for the therapist...

...not really knowing HOW to progress a patient...

...or second-guessing if that patient is ready to return to the higher loading activities...

...questioning when to progress them or even if they are being aggressive enough with the rehab.

This lack of confidence and clarity shows up as a lack of authority from the therapist. The patient then loses confidence in them, doesn't adhere to the exercises and soon stalls in progress. Eventually, they are polite to the therapist, make some excuse and drop off.

This lack of clinical reasoning and a common sense step-by-step progressive approach is costing therapists their reputation and recognition but also thousands upon thousands of pounds in RETENTION, REFERRALS, REVENUE and even job opportunities.

Save yourself years and learn from my mistakes

In this book, I'll share my mistakes so you can learn from them. I'll also share the exact method I used in the 2017 Rugby League World Cup final week to rule in one player and rule out our most influential player and how I knew I made the right decision.

I'll also share how I get patients to return consistently to my own private practice even if it has been years since they last came, how my client base has spread by word of mouth even though our fees are much higher than every other physio clinic around us and how I've grown my clinic from a one treatment room, one-man clinic to now having five treatment rooms, a yoga studio and ten staff with a practice manager overseeing it all so I still get paid and make money while on holiday with my family.

All you need is an open mind and to be ready to see and hear.

CHAPTER 2
My road to success

My very first job was at Leeds Rhinos and Yorkshire Carnegie (Leeds Carnegie at the time), in a split role initially, before moving over full time to the Rhinos the following season.

My very first injury to treat was an ankle syndesmosis injury and I remember thinking to myself 'What the heck is a syndesmosis injury?' I had never heard of that or certainly couldn't remember covering it in university, although, in all honesty, we may well have done.

But as any good therapist does at times, I winged it with the utmost confidence (joking!) and luckily didn't mess up the patient in that session before I could grab five minutes and look up what the actual injury meant.

I've had a case where a player had a recurrent hamstring tear where I'd promised the coach he'd be good to return to playing for the weekend and he actually re-injured his hamstring the day before his expected returning to training because I truly didn't understand the importance of a progressive step-by-step plan and where the athlete was in that plan.

I've been fortunate enough (if you want to look at it that way) to have been exposed to some of the most complex knee injuries you will see and have had the opportunity to rehab them from start to finish.

[You can watch Danny McGuire's multi-ligament reconstruction video at this resource: www.thegotophysiobook.com/resources]

I was very fortunate to have had a great mentor at Leeds Rhinos in Meirion Jones who helped me develop a very strong hands-on treatment approach and allowed me to really see the value of strength work (at the right time) and how important it was for the athlete to lift well in the gym.

Around this time, I was just setting up my own private practice in

Huddersfield, forming a company called ProSport Physiotherapy with Meirion and another one of my mentors, Martin Higgins, who I was really lucky to learn from while on my final student placement at Bradford Bulls.

I was growing the Huddersfield clinic myself, doing it the hard way relying on word-of-mouth referrals from downstairs and the few people I knew in the town. But the results were gaining momentum and I was quickly making some nice revenue and enjoying the retention and referrals, based solely on word of mouth from happy past patients.

When I left for Munster, I thought I was well on my way to becoming that Go-To Therapist. We split the clinics in ProSport Physiotherapy with me keeping the Huddersfield clinic. I had a good young therapist looking after the clinic while I offered him mentorship with weekly calls and sorted him an internship with one of my good friends who was now head physio at Bradford Bulls.

Sure, I had some great results at Munster, as I did with Leeds, but I had two players retire on my watch due to injury which led to a sour taste in my mouth and a harsh awakening to reality that I was far from being the finished product.

It was great, however, to work in a different organisation and get the opportunity to work with so many excellent Strength and Conditioning Coaches at Munster who all brought something unique to the table.

This really helped me to look at the WHOLE body and the whole journey of the patient or athlete.

When I got approached by Huddersfield Giants to lead their medical team, it was a no-brainer as my wife (fiancée at the time), Georgina, and Ava who was two and a half were still in Huddersfield and reluctant to move to Ireland.

This was then a great opportunity for me to implement a complete injury prevention strategy that was a hybrid of what we were doing with Leeds and Munster but also to finally right some wrongs and develop a sound, clinically reasoned step-by-step approach.

I sat down and listed my strengths and weaknesses from every aspect of the patient journey from subjective assessment, to pain neuroscience education, to hands-on treatment, to rehab, to S and C, and scored myself out of ten.

I then focused my attention on the lowest scores to get them up to par while also implementing and integrating everything together as a system. I used the Huddersfield Giants as my private laboratory as I had the advantage of access to players pretty much as and when I wanted to see them.

This proved massively beneficial in seeing the LONG-TERM EFFECTS of the input I was applying to their nervous system. I quickly became tired of short-term quick fixes that didn't stick.

This was when it really dawned on me that if I was to input into my patient's nervous system via whatever means – words, hands-on, rehab – then the protective REACTIONS for the vast majority of cases should disappear.

So, then, rather than fixing the first thing I saw on the bed or in my assessment, I started asking myself the higher level questions covered in Chapter 1. This led me to working SMARTER not HARDER and I found I was doing a lot less hands-on treatment and then had the time with the athlete to do the exercises and make progress.

I then focused on creating a logical, step-by-step progressive method from the bed to the field, and in the last two years I have really worked hard on drilling this down to the last detail so as to ensure a smooth transition back to play.

My clarity and confidence exploded and I found it much easier to tell the coach when the player would be back training and to justify it logically. By the time Ruby Rae, my second daughter, arrived I knew my time in full-time sport was limited.

I was receiving more and more emails from therapists I had got to know over the years asking me clinical questions and I was also shocked at how poorly prepared final year physiotherapy students were for the real world so I decided to set up an online website called

www.theprosportacademy.com.

From here, in 2015, I developed the Online Therapist Mentorship just for fun to see if there would be any interest and was amazed that 25 people signed up.

The clinic was also growing nicely and I had a full-time therapist, Shane Mooney, doing a great job working for me there so I was confident I could increase my private practice caseload to make up the salary I'd be missing from the Giants.

The Giants tried to keep me on the books consulting formally but we eventually came to a casual arrangement which allowed me more time to focus on the Online Mentorship.

When I left the Giants at the end of 2015, I honestly thought I'd do one or two mentorships and this would give me some time to build the practice up. To my surprise the mentorship grew faster than the clinic and I realised there were many other therapists out there who were going through similar problems and challenges that I had gone through.

As I continued to refine the system, especially in private practice, I found my own confidence and clarity continued to improve and the results were getting even more consistent and predictable. I decided to continue with the Online Mentorship and I'm proud to say I've now got over two hundred therapists worldwide implementing the content and making a meaningful impact on patients' lives where traditional approaches have failed.

The extra time I had out of full-time sport allowed me to consult with other professional clubs and athletes in addition to the clinical caseload I had taken on. I was continuing to learn more and more and gaining even more clarity as to WHY my system was working for me as I knew I had an obligation to justify each step which really made me ask myself some serious questions.

At the start of 2017, England Rugby League came knocking on my door. I'd rejected the opportunity to work with them on two occasions in the past, but the time and situation was finally right for me. The step-by-step approach again proved invaluable during the World Cup in Australia and New Zealand.

I enjoyed a relatively stress-free time during the World Cup and I put that down to having the step-by-step approach in place which helped me make logical decisions rather than emotional decisions, as can so easily happen in sport.

Currently, I am dividing my time between consulting and mentoring Warrington Wolves Head Physiotherapist one day a week, working for the England Rugby League position and other professional sports athletes, teaching on my mentorship, mentoring my own therapists in my clinic and seeing a case of patients that have complex histories and failed traditional approaches.

The step-by-step approach has evolved massively, even since leaving the Giants in 2015. The thought process and the principles are the same but the movements, hands-on treatment and even neuroscience education has just become so much easier, and more logical and straightforward.

I have never worked as easily as I do now with less hands-on treatment than ever before and more exercises within sessions that solve a patient's problem to progress them to the next level.

Everything I do has purpose, clarity and reasoning and the results have been even more consistent and predictable, not just for me, but for my therapists in my clinic. Everything I teach in my Online Mentorship is REAL WORLD information that we use on a daily basis and that can be applied in the real world.

What I am about to share with you now is the result of ten-plus years of making mistakes, learning from them, and refining and repeating this process.

CHAPTER 3
Could we be looking at things from the wrong side?

Could we be looking at the solution to the patient's problem the wrong way around? Could there be more than just thinking: 'Here's a person in pain; I need to decrease the pain experience and load the painful tissues around the painful site'?

Is doing this simply treating the *reaction* to the pain experience?

What caused the peripheral tissues to be overloaded in the first place?

What contributed to an even greater pain experience centrally (and/or peripherally)?

What about if the Go-To Therapist asked WHY is that tissue irritated or overloaded in the first place? Why is the person having an unpleasant perception about THIS AREA of the body?

What would happen to that pain experience if we found which areas were not contributing enough and got these areas doing their job again?

Would this be a quicker, more efficient and longer-lasting way of working for both the therapist and patient?

Would this help take the pain experience away quicker? I'm not sure and I don't claim to have all the answers but these are just some of the questions going through my mind each time I assess a patient.

The Go-To Therapist doesn't accept dated explanations or the old-fashioned statement: 'it's just one of those things'.

They are energised, enthused and hungry for knowledge and information. They question every injury, make the most of every opportunity to learn lessons from the failures in the system at present and constantly work out how they can do things better.

The Go-To Therapists in my Online Mentorship have been made aware of certain things that to the best of my knowledge are based on the most up-to-date literature at the time of writing. These have had a massive influence on my approach.

The Go-To Therapist:

- **Understands that pain is an output of the brain and does not simply mean damage to a tissue**

The Go-To Therapist understands that pain is a conscious experience and simply an output of the brain.

The Go-To Therapist educates his/her patients on what pain is and what it is not via effective explanation to give the patient the best chance of understanding and doesn't simply throw random terms at the patient without any relevance to them or their story.

 The Go-To Therapist chooses their words carefully and does not simply use lazy language that ultimately may come back to haunt them later.

They explain things in a way that is meaningful to the patient so they can understand why their body may be organising itself in this way and why they are experiencing these unpleasant conscious sensations of pain, tightness etc.

The Go-To Therapist knows that there are many facets to the pain output experience and it is ultimately an interpretation from the body and brain from actual or 'perceived threats' to the system.

They use this knowledge to their advantage when managing acute injuries/ presentations to reassure patients. This will ultimately help decrease the protective reactions.

- *Understands that stress precedes pain and can come in many forms*

The Go-To Therapist appreciates the role of stress or stressors on the body.

They appreciate that many things can act as stressors such as compensation strategies still in place due to previous injuries; emotional stressors placed on athletes/patients as a result of team sporting environments; work, contracts and family issues.

The Go-To Therapist understands that tissues such as the diaphragm and pelvic floor may react to such stressors with protective tone and this can then influence the movement variability of the athlete.

They appreciate that stressors such as diet, sleep and other lifestyle choices can impact our breathing rate, our ability to recover and variability between our heart rate, breathing rate and movement.

They appreciate how emotional and lifestyle stressors can alter the tone of the diaphragm and pelvic floor in anticipation to perceived threats or repeated bouts of trauma on the body such as contact training or sporting activities or specific events/environments/places for the non-sporting patient.

They appreciate the importance of the diaphragm and pelvic floor's ability to lengthen and shorten in order to maintain movement variability, and how emotional and lifestyle stressors may have an influence on a patient's movement options.

They appreciate that in the same way that nociceptors can become sensitised, so too can the chemoreceptors. This can affect the depth of our breathing which will affect the amplitude of diaphragm and pelvic floor movement and indirectly hence affect the musculoskeletal system such as thoracic mobility or pelvic mobility.

- *Understands that noxious stimulus can alter directions of force*

The Go-To Therapist understands that when there is a noxious stimulus to the system (think dead leg or bump to the leg in sport) the body goes about organising itself to be successful for that moment in time.

They understand that the patient/athlete may not even have a conscious awareness of the subtle differences in how their system has organised itself but their movement strategies will have altered as a result.

They understand this could be significant when tracing back previous injuries and making sense of the objective assessment or how the patient/athlete is moving now.

They will respect the injury history and the nervous system's attempts to keep the patient/athlete successful in their sporting environment but understand that there may be a long-term consequence of such strategy for the athlete on other tissues or joints which may have become sensitised.

They will understand the value in restoring and reassuring the patient/athlete's belief system in generating torque in particular directions and having the intent to produce force in as many options as possible.

They will use this understanding to their advantage throughout the treatment plan.

- *Understands the generic reactions of the body to parasympathetic dominance*

The Go-To Therapist appreciates that movement 'dysfunctions' or 'compensations' are simply strategies in reaction to pain or parasympathetic dominance and not the true cause.

They understand that the patient will attempt to succeed by using strategies such as excessively elevating the ribcage to overcome muscle slack in the mid-section.

They understand that patients in parasympathetic dominance will favour mouth breathing, will have decreased amplitude of the diaphragm and pelvic floor during respiration (which may or may not influence decreased movement variability), and decreased variance of movement through the full foot when moving both in the gym and when decelerating.

They understand that how the patient's body will self-organise will be entirely unique to that patient and the true stressor is unique to them even though they may seem to move in similar ways to other patients.

The Go-To Therapist will strive to find the true stressors no matter what system they are working with and will no longer tolerate just treating the site of the issue and hoping for the best.

The Go-To Therapist understands that sometimes the true stressor is not physical but there is still plenty that they can do to manage the overreactions of the system within their scope of practice.

The above are some of my beliefs and thoughts at the moment based on my interpretation and understanding of the literature. For further reading on these areas, please visit www.thegotophysiobook.com/resources

The other question on my mind is whether pathology, time frames, textbooks and surgeons are limiting our beliefs and abilities as clinicians.

As many rugby league and union physiotherapists will attest to, some patients/athletes who have quite a lot of pathology on scans are moving around pain-free and without a care in the world while other patients/athletes with minimal pathology are reported to be in all sorts of pain.

The Go-To Therapist understands WHY there is a difference here and the need to consider other stressors.

For example, I've had numerous players playing with high grade MCL tears that are 'functionally' stable. Indeed I followed the advice of an orthopaedic surgeon in Melbourne who recommended not bracing an MCL. I did my job, took the player through a graded exposure, and he did extremely well.

I have also had a large number of athletes and private practice patients diagnosed with SLAP tears who were able to make a full 'functional' recovery.
Although post-op instructions, especially with regards to healing times, need to be respected, when we progress people logically through a step-by-step progressive pathway, the results can be amazing. These progressions

are made logically rather than emotionally and the patient has earned the right to progress; but more on how you do this later.

I also believe that in a profession such as physiotherapy we need to be slower to dismiss WHY something is working because of a lack of hard evidence but rather ask better questions and attempt to answer these through research, the best we can.

Finally, on this topic, I believe there is a desperate need for research that will help clinicians improve their clinical reasoning in the real world. For example there was a paper by Scarfe et al in 2011 that is extremely useful in helping therapists put together a step-by-step progressive programme, yet there have only been three citations of this paper since with no follow-up.

But anyway, enough of the WHAT IFS and let's get down to the nitty gritty of the Go-To Therapist Method in the next chapter.

CHAPTER 4
The Go-To Therapist Method overview

So let's get started IMPLEMENTING in the real world! If you know anything about me by now, you'll know that I pride myself in the fact that everything I deliver you can implement in the real world.

The five critical clinical components to ensuring you build a word-of-mouth reputation/clinic that allows you to raise your Revenue, Rates, Referrals and Recognition by getting great Results are:

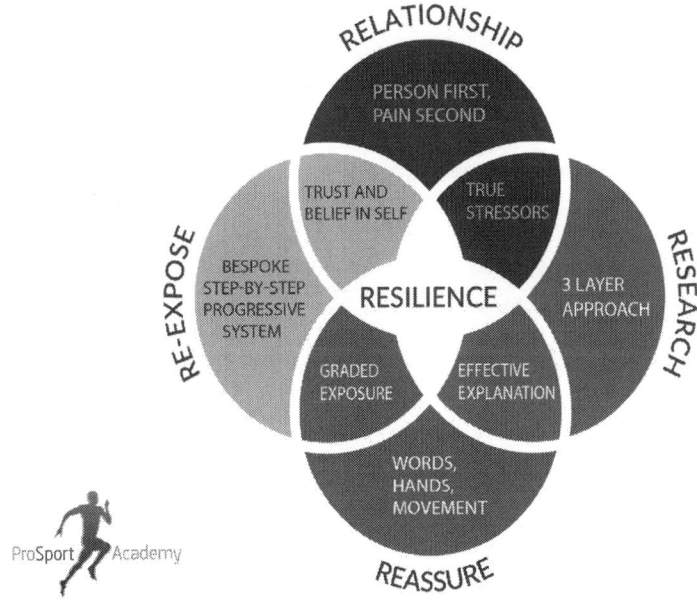

This is the bird's eye view so you can gain a quick insight into what's to follow in more detail in the coming chapters. But for now let's visit each component briefly.

1 RELATIONSHIP

The first component to ensuring great, long-lasting, consistent results is RELATIONSHIP.

Whether you are comfortable hearing this or not, you need to develop a relationship with the patient and build a CONNECTION in the first session.

If you build a CONNECTION with your patient and they feel listened to and understood this will be worth much more than attending ten hands-on treatment courses I promise.

There will ALWAYS be a reason for someone's pain or trauma to a tissue such as a hamstring tear. And, from my experience with non-traumatic injuries, it is NEVER 'just because the tissue was weak'. Ultimately it was the tissue's capacity to tolerate load that was exceeded that eventually led to this trauma.

BUT WHY?

For a persistent back or neck pain patient, there may be other non-physical contributors to the pain experience.

It is YOUR JOB as a therapist to make sense of the story and find the 'true stressors' that caused the tissue to exceed its capacity in the first place. The answer will always lie in the story and can be found from a combination of the following three stressors:

- **Physical Stressors**
- **Emotional Stressors**
- **Lifestyle Stressors**

If you can make sense of the story and start to build a working hypothesis, then this allows you to make sense of the objective assessment enabling you to identify potential tripwires that may be overlooked further down the line that would contribute to setbacks or flare-ups.

In order for the patient to trust you and offer this personal and sometimes upsetting information, we need to build connections in this Patient-Therapist RELATIONSHIP.

2 RESEARCH

Now that you have an understanding and a potential working hypothesis of the numerous factors contributing to this painful experience, it is time to RESEARCH which peripheral tissues may be contributing to the pain experience, if any, either directly or indirectly via motor adaptations from previous injuries, or as a reaction to stress in general.

While traditionally we were taught (or certainly I was taught) to focus on the site of the pain, to load it and strengthen it, the Go-To Therapist is looking for areas of the body that are NOT doing enough!

Rather than focusing 80% of your time trying to strengthen tissues that have more than likely been overloaded or overworked in the first place, you are going to spend 80% of your time focusing on the tissues that are NOT doing their job so the sensitised tissues can actually do less, not more work when back in the real world.

The part of the movement that the pain experience occurs can give you clues as to what peripheral tissues may be contributing to the pain experience at this moment or more importantly **what tissues ARE NOT contributing towards the movement efficiently which may result in other tissues having to absorb the movement errors synergistically.** This information combined with traditional assessments such as your passive joint assessment and other tests will give you clues as to how the body has responded to that person's story.

By the end of your second component you should have clarity on the next steps that will have your attention broken down into an 80/20 style.

20% of your attention, time and energy will be spent on the peripheral tissues (if any) directly contributing to the pain experience (for example, a painful tendon may undergo some loading protocol).

80% of your attention, time and energy will be spent on the peripheral tissues not doing enough work and the non-physical contributors that are contributing to the pain experience specific to that person's story and based on your research. (For example, your research found that a previous hamstring injury was affecting the ability of the knee to co-contract so the quadriceps were doing excessive work and sending high loads to the tendon. Therefore 80% of your attention, time and energy in treatment and rehab is focused on restoring the ability of the knee to co-contract when decelerating.)

From my experience, this will ensure that once the patient returns to the real world the true stressors have been addressed and the symptoms will not return again.

3 REASSURANCE

You are now ready to start the treatment plan and the first step is REASSURANCE.

Reassurance can come in many ways including education, hands-on treatment and non-manual therapy techniques.

The first step in the Go-To Therapist Mentorship is via effective explanation. Rather than overwhelm the patient with lots of new words and medical terms, we keep things simple so **the person can understand the PROBLEM rather than just have a DIAGNOSIS.**

If a person understands the problem, then the next logical
step is to find out the solution

(In the example above, the diagnosis would be a Patella Tendonosis but the problem is that the hamstring is not working efficiently under isometric-like conditions due to a previous hamstring injury, so the quadriceps are working excessively when decelerating.)

If the person understands the problem, they will then be clear on WHY they are doing an exercise to allow the hamstring an opportunity to work under isometric-like conditions again and, from my experience, you will have a far greater chance of patient adherence. The reassurance will continue in the form of hands-on treatment.

However in the Go-To Therapist approach, the hands-on treatment is not some evil tool, as sadly some are claiming in our profession these days, but rather it interlinks with two components of the Go-To Therapist Method: Reassurance and Re-Exposure.

The hands-on treatment is the starting point to RE-EXPOSING the tissues we've RESEARCHED that are not doing enough for the person to tolerate load again, but it is done in a very REASSURING manner.

The intention is not to break up scar tissue or anything like that with our hands-on treatment but to simply REASSURE the nervous system it is safe to tolerate load in the direction you've identified in the assessment.

4 RE-EXPOSURE

The fourth component in the Go-To Therapist Method is to RE-EXPOSE the tissues that are not contributing enough to the movement you've identified from your RESEARCH and to continue to REASSURE these tissues and the person's nervous system to tolerate loading at each level.

A new level of load to tolerate; a new problem for the
nervous system to figure out

From my experience of working with hundreds of pro athletes especially, once you expose the person's tissues and nervous system to new levels of loading, new problems start to appear.

So in this step, the ProSport Academy 'Return To Loading Step-By-Step Progressions' really comes to the fore where the next progression is the next logical step.

This does not mean that just because a person is pain free doing a lunge in the treatment room for example, that they are safe to now return to higher loading activities such as running. The Go-To Therapist understands that they need to expose the person's nervous system to higher levels of stress on the peripheral tissues but also at higher speeds of contraction that happen at similar ground reaction forces that the person will need to tolerate to be successful in everyday life.

Therefore you RE-EXPOSE your patient in a logical step-by-step manner, understanding WHEN and HOW to progress the patient so they continue to make progress in every single session.

The Go-To Therapist exposes the person's nervous system to similar loads and actually supra-maximally exposes the tissues that originally were not contributing enough in the first place. They then observe closely for any reactions such as loss of joint range of motion, swelling or whatever key performance indicators they will be using with this patient. If there are no negative reactions then the therapist can be very confident the person is now ready to return to these tasks in the real world.

5. RESILIENCE

When you put all these R's together, something magical happens for the patient. Because you have built a relationship with the patient and researched, reassured and re-exposed them to MEANINGFUL activities that add value to their life, their self-confidence grows massively and you can now discharge them with a plan to further build resilience to both physical and mental loads that they will be exposed to in real life.

And when you can add so much value to a patient's life like this and operate on this level of expertise, the patient actually wants their friends and family to experience the same transformations and so will actively go out of their way to promote you and your business, helping you become the Go-To Therapist.

If you can achieve consistently great results and every patient refers you to at least two others DUE TO THE RESULTS, then you will have a very busy practice quickly.

This is why I believe having the confidence, clarity and structure to get consistently great results is the quickest and cheapest way to Rapidly Raise your Retention, Rates, Revenues, Referrals and Recognition as the Go-To Therapist.

Word-of-mouth Referrals is the Quickest and Cheapest Way to Build a Sustainable Profitable Business

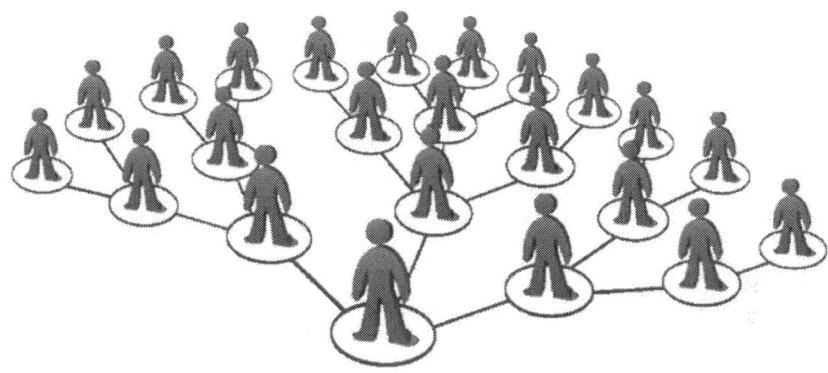

Be the guide not the hero

Before I break this down into 12 easy steps for you, it is important to remember that at all times you are the GUIDE and NOT THE HERO. Make this story and transformation about the patient.

Resist the urge to say 'I did this or I did that' with your hands-on treatment or rehab. Instead an approach where 'I just helped YOUR nervous system to tolerate loading of these tissues a little better and now you will continue to reassure it further with these simple exercises' brings it all back to the person rather than you physically doing something, such as breaking up scar tissue for instance.

Keep your language clean and simple.

And with that said, in the next chapter, let's break these 5 critical components down into 12 simple steps that you can use in the real world.

What Go-To Therapists had to say about the mentorship

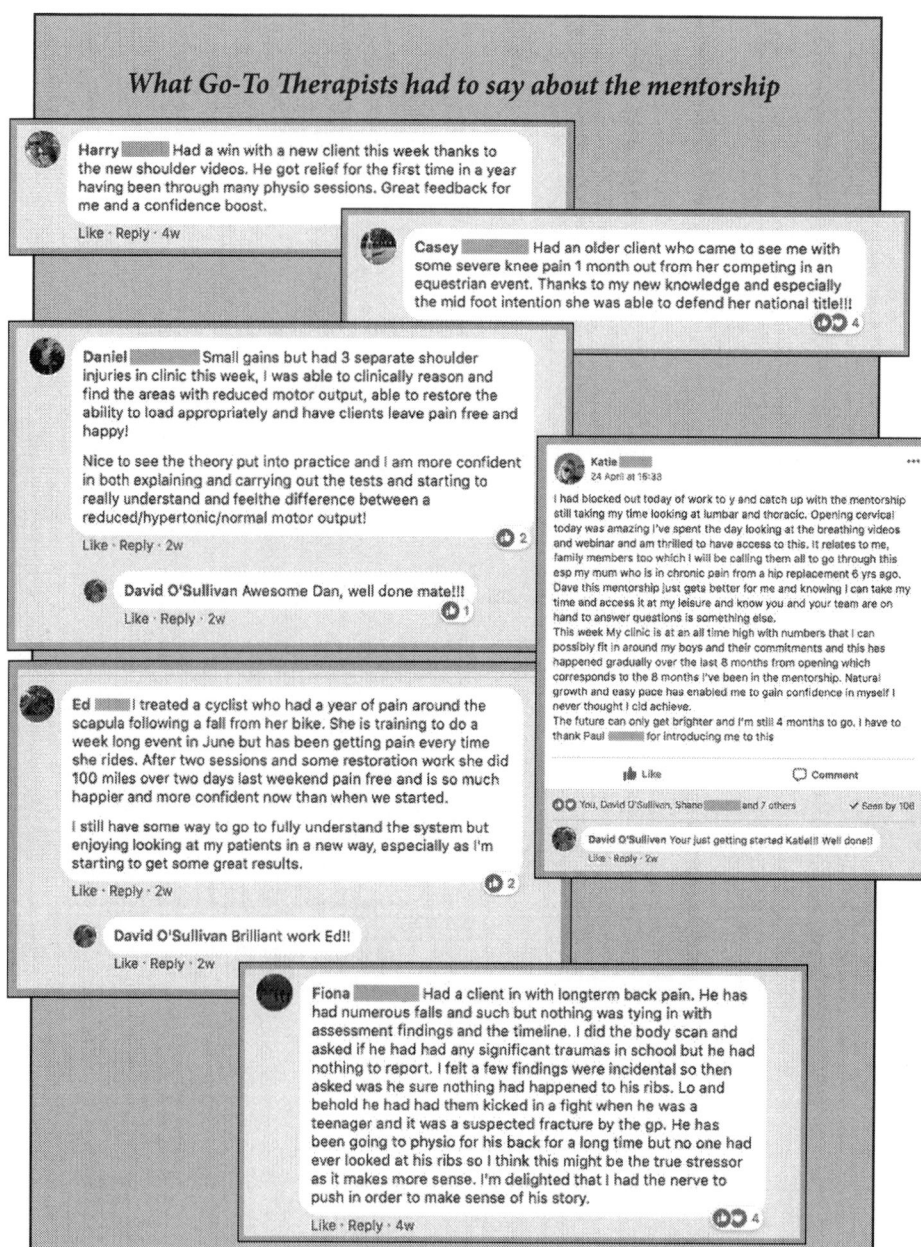

Harry ▨▨▨ Had a win with a new client this week thanks to the new shoulder videos. He got relief for the first time in a year having been through many physio sessions. Great feedback for me and a confidence boost.

Like · Reply · 4w

Casey ▨▨▨ Had an older client who came to see me with some severe knee pain 1 month out from her competing in an equestrian event. Thanks to my new knowledge and especially the mid foot intention she was able to defend her national title!!!

Daniel ▨▨▨ Small gains but had 3 separate shoulder injuries in clinic this week, I was able to clinically reason and find the areas with reduced motor output, able to restore the ability to load appropriately and have clients leave pain free and happy!

Nice to see the theory put into practice and I am more confident in both explaining and carrying out the tests and starting to really understand and feel the difference between a reduced/hypertonic/normal motor output!

Like · Reply · 2w

> **David O'Sullivan** Awesome Dan, well done mate!!!
> Like · Reply · 2w

Katie ▨▨▨
24 April at 15:33

I had blocked out today of work to y and catch up with the mentorship still taking my time looking at lumbar and thoracic. Opening cervical today was amazing I've spent the day looking at the breathing videos and webinar and am thrilled to have access to this. It relates to me, family members too which I will be calling them all to go through this esp my mum who is in chronic pain from a hip replacement 6 yrs ago. Dave this mentorship just gets better for me and knowing I can take my time and access it at my leisure and know you and your team are on hand to answer questions is something else.
This week My clinic is at an all time high with numbers that I can possibly fit in around my boys and their commitments and this has happened gradually over the last 8 months from opening which corresponds to the 8 months I've been in the mentorship. Natural growth and easy pace has enabled me to gain confidence in myself I never thought I cld achieve.
The future can only get brighter and I'm still 4 months to go. I have to thank Paul ▨▨▨ for introducing me to this

👍 Like   💬 Comment

You, David O'Sullivan, Shane ▨▨▨ and 7 others   ✓ Seen by 108

> **David O'Sullivan** Your just getting started Katie!!! Well done!!
> Like · Reply · 2w

Ed ▨▨▨ I treated a cyclist who had a year of pain around the scapula following a fall from her bike. She is training to do a week long event in June but has been getting pain every time she rides. After two sessions and some restoration work she did 100 miles over two days last weekend pain free and is so much happier and more confident now than when we started.

I still have some way to go to fully understand the system but enjoying looking at my patients in a new way, especially as I'm starting to get some great results.

Like · Reply · 2w

> **David O'Sullivan** Brilliant work Ed!!
> Like · Reply · 2w

Fiona ▨▨▨ Had a client in with longterm back pain. He has had numerous falls and such but nothing was tying in with assessment findings and the timeline. I did the body scan and asked if he had had any significant traumas in school but he had nothing to report. I felt a few findings were incidental so then asked was he sure nothing had happened to his ribs. Lo and behold he had had them kicked in a fight when he was a teenager and it was a suspected fracture by the gp. He has been going to physio for his back for a long time but no one had ever looked at his ribs so I think this might be the true stressor as it makes more sense. I'm delighted that I had the nerve to push in order to make sense of his story.

Like · Reply · 4w

CHAPTER 5
Step 1 Making sense of your patient's story and having confidence and clarity in your treatment plan

Your first job in the initial assessment is to make your patient feel at ease and comfortable. They need to get used to you, your voice, the environment and many other things.

Asking them some simple questions about the immediate past such as 'Did you find us OK?' to start with is a great way to get them used to listening to your voice and answering questions.

I then like to set the scene in the initial assessment to tell the patient exactly what they can expect in this session. This will hopefully put them further at ease and eliminate the 'fear of the unknown' which can be very real for some patients. It also creates authority for you in that you are leading/guiding the session and all future sessions.

Once you've got the patient settled, the biggest mistake I see being made is to focus all yours and your patient's attention on their 'pain'.

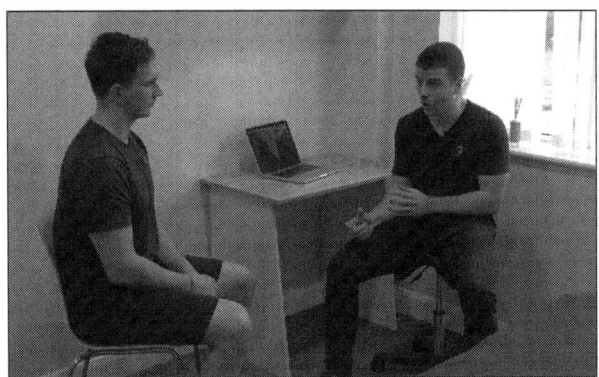

All questions are usually about the pain: scoring the pain, getting the pain's 24-hour pattern etc., etc. Instead forget about that traditional method for the moment and imagine you had ten minutes to get to know this person and actively listen to them with interest about how their story and how this pain is affecting THEIR LIFE.

Now the person's attention (and yours) is all on them and it is about *them* rather than the pain.

You are listening for clues and genuinely trying to make sense from their story as to why this pain experience is present in the first place.

There will ALWAYS be a reason for someone's pain or trauma to a tissue such as a hamstring tear or back pain. And, from my experience with non-traumatic injuries, it is NEVER 'just because the tissue was weak'.

Ultimately it was the tissue's capacity to tolerate load that was exceeded that eventually led to this trauma.

BUT WHY?

It is your job as a therapist to make sense of the story and find the 'true stressors' that caused the tissue to exceed its capacity in the first place.

The answer will always lie in the story and can be found from a combination of the following three stressors using the 'Stressor and Story Method':

- **Physical Stressors (Previous injuries and motor adaptations to pain or noxious stimuli)**

- **Emotional Stressors (Motor adaptations in the musculoskeletal system as a result of a sensitised respiratory system among other adaptations)**

- **Lifestyle Stressors (Adaptations in various systems of the body as a result of excessive stressors due to lifestyle such as sleep and diet)**

Now most patients will want to talk straight away about their pain, just like most therapists, but the Go-To Therapist will want to make sense of this and be very interested in previous injuries, events and significant periods of stress prior to the pain experience becoming present.

Most patients will dismiss previous injuries away from the site of pain as irrelevant but it's your job to find these and ask the logical question: could any of these injuries adapt/change the patient's movement behaviour and potentially overload the area where the patient is now experiencing pain?

Obviously, it goes without saying, you must clear your red flags and special questions but the point I'm making is to get to know your patient and their story rather than just the site of pain.

This will be invaluable information in the next step when we look at the generic objective assessment and make sense of how the person's nervous system has adapted to their story.

The final bit of information you need to elicit is where the patient wants to get back to – and don't just accept 'to get out of pain' as an answer.

Having a deep understanding of the activities that add value to their life is very important as this will now direct YOUR attention on which direction the treatment plan will go in when implemented once you have made sense of how the person's body has adapted and self-organised in response to their previous injuries and stressors.

In the Go-To Therapist Online Mentorship, we pride ourselves on asking high quality questions to get meaningful information that can be put to work straight away. I'd encourage you to do so too.

CHAPTER 6
Step 2 Making sense of the objective assessment

Now that you have a sense of understanding and a potential working hypothesis of the numerous factors contributing to the patient's painful experience, it is time to narrow down which peripheral tissues may be contributing to the pain experience, if any.

We use the 'three-layer approach' in the objective assessment to gain clarity on what needs 'undoing' to help with the symptoms and what we must help the patient get back, to ensure that the problem does not return again.

The 'three-layer approach' includes:

- **Generic Objective Assessment**
- **Passive Assessment**
- **Directions Of Force Production Coordination Testing**

The value in using the 'three-layer approach' above, in addition to the 'Stressor and Story Method' in the subjective assessment, is that as you progress through the assessment you are building a stronger and stronger hypothesis of where to start your treatment plan.

The REAL VALUE, however, is that if you have missed something in either the subjective assessment or one of the layers, then the other layers don't usually make sense as you progress through the objective assessment, and so you won't end up on a wild goose chase, taking your patient's rehab plan in the wrong direction.

APPLIED EXAMPLE

A really quick example of this happened to me personally when working with a professional golfer a few years' back. The patient came to see me with a right-sided meniscal tear that was stable and he was managing OK until the end of the season. In his history he was only ever mentioning his right side (an old ankle sprain) and denied any issues with his left leg.

There was no known mechanism for the knee pain and it came on gradually so I was really struggling to make sense of why this happened and was presuming it may have been down to adaptations laid down by the previous ankle injury. As we headed for the objective assessment, I still wasn't comfortable with having made sense of his story but we proceeded anyway.

In the objective assessment, he was very protective of his LEFT leg subconsciously from what I saw in the generic assessment which again didn't make sense with his story. I kept probing him for anything at all that happened on his left leg which he continued to deny.

The next layer, the passive assessment, gave me a better clue about the symptoms and range of motion on both sides but there was nothing remarkable.

It was only when I was putting him on his side for the final part of the objective assessment that I noticed an old scar on the side of his LEFT knee. I asked him about this and he said it happened when he was about eight and he fell backwards through his patio doors in his living room.

The final layer then revealed that he really struggled to coordinate and generate force submaximally in certain directions on this left leg. So now this was starting to make sense and also correlated nicely with what he felt was happening in his golf swing and what his golf coach was trying to achieve with him.

So now I was a lot happier with making sense of the story and working on a hypothesis that there was a protective response or 'perceived threat' still present from the nervous system with regards tolerating loads in certain directions on the LEFT leg.

The treatment plan was also a lot clearer for both of us with some hands-on treatment to desensitise the right knee (20% of my attention) but the majority of my attention (80%) with my rehab would focus on helping the patient reassure his nervous system that it was not only safe to tolerate load at low levels but also high loads at high speeds on his left leg, which we will discuss in further chapters.

Although it is not essential for peripheral tissues to be involved in a painful experience, it is my experience that there will be some involvement from the peripheral tissues towards the pain experience in most injuries, either directly or indirectly via motor adaptations from previous injuries, or as a reaction to stress in general.

The Generic Objective Assessment is now an opportunity for your patient to do some simple 'big' movements like touching their toes, bending backwards etc and to gain an appreciation of how they are achieving these tasks WITHOUT trying to diagnose based on just these few movements.

This is the starting point of the objective assessment; we need to go through the other two layers to further strengthen our working hypothesis of the true problem.

In my Go-To Therapist Mentorship, I do not actively cue or look for 'ideal' movements. What I am looking for mainly is that the movement is done with 'thoughtless, fearless movement' (a term coined by the late Louis Gifford) and that they are happy to challenge their base of support subconsciously.

The part of the movement where the pain experience occurs can give you clues as to what peripheral tissues may be contributing to the pain experience at this moment or more importantly what tissues ARE NOT contributing towards the movement efficiently which may result in other tissues having to absorb the movement errors synergistically.

Other clues may be in the form of what the person IS NOT loading in these basic movements. The patient may look over their right shoulder and twist their whole body in this direction and you might notice that they are not putting much weight on the right heel.

Now the right heel may not be the problem; the problem may be that by putting weight through that right heel they are putting a load on certain tissues such as the biceps femoris, for example. Is there a subconscious movement behaviour of avoiding loading an old hamstring injury or of loading certain fibres of muscles as a motor adaptation to pain or a previous noxious stimulus?

Again, this is a working hypothesis and so we would need to make sense of this in the patient's story and also further justify our hypothesis as we progress through the objective assessment.

APPLIED EXAMPLE

A classic example of this is the toe touch test used by many therapists where at the start of the movement the patient experiences pain in the low back region, similar to a disc-type or SIJ-type presentation.

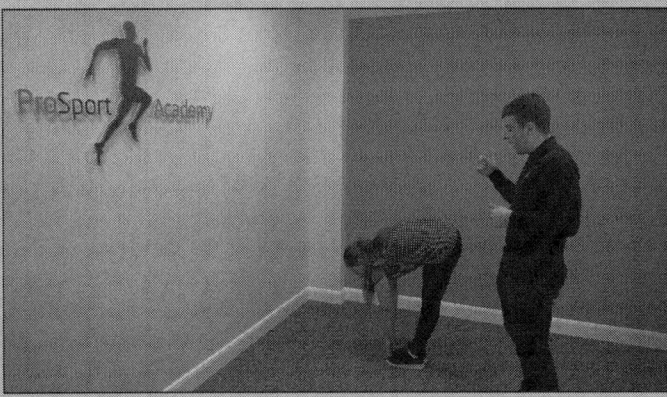

The low back tissues should not be the main ones absorbing the load at this point of the movement and should be starting to relax as the ribcage depresses while the person's fingertips lead the movement of touching their toes.

An inability of the ribcage to depress proficiently, the diaphragm to lengthen and the pelvic floor to ascend in the initial movement may contribute to the iliocostalis tissues, for example, absorbing the errors and additional load in the movement which may contribute to the pain experience.

The iliocostalis tissues have tendons inserted onto the rib cage and so, as the person's rib cage depresses anteriorly, the posterior tissues, including the myotendinous junctions of the iliocostalis, lengthen and relax the muscle.

If the person is stiff through the ribcage and not moving it well due to a sensitised respiratory system as a result of ongoing non-physical stressors, could we now be seeing the result of this in the physical form with an adaptation in movement behaviour?

If the iliocostalis tissues are not lengthening but are actually contracting now, is this causing a prediction error for the nervous system? The majority of the load from these tissues generating force will naturally go towards the insertion which just so happens to be around the low back area and the thoracic lumbar fascia.

If a nerve is suddenly getting irritated or a disc is becoming sensitised, could this be as a result of a reaction from the iliocostalis, as a result of a reaction from a sensitised respiratory system due to the stressor specific to that individual?

Obviously, I appreciate this is a theory and working hypothesis as I mentioned, and the iliocostalis may be one such tissue to adapt.

However, remember: clinical reasoning is king and you can cross-reference your working hypothesis with different movements to further check your work.

For example, if you believed the lack of lengthening of the diaphragm (as a result of adaptations of a sensitised respiratory system perhaps) was a major contributor to the pain experience, then you may not expect to see the patient experience pain with a backward bend where the rib cage would be elevating and the diaphragm would not be required to lengthen but to actually shorten.

Therefore rather than just jumping to assumptions based on one movement, the Go-To Therapist continues to clinically reason as they progress through the assessment.

At this point of the assessment, you are still only hypothesising and linking together how the respiratory system and the inability of the diaphragm to go through a full range of motion (as research has suggested in those undergoing prolonged stress) may be contributing to movement inefficiency which is ultimately resulting in a pain experience for the person.

There would be further clues in the next two sections of the objective assessment for this particular back pain case that would further strengthen our working hypothesis and would lead to some quick and easy ways to intervene and retest.

There are clues everywhere in the objective assessment and sometimes we just need to unravel these adaptations but first and foremost we need to understand the patient's story as shown in the previous step.

The next step in the 'three-layer approach' is the passive assessment which can add so much more valuable information to the working hypothesis with some sound clinical reasoning.

CHAPTER 7

Step 3 How to know where to start with your hands-on treatment

So now you have an idea of some peripheral tissues that are contributing to the pain experience that would make sense from the subjective story also, it is time to find some further adaptations laid down by the nervous system. Before we get into the passive assessment, one of my biggest pieces of advice that I want to give you, which was a game changer for me, is to avoid treating the first adaptation you see.

For example, if there is decreased hip flexion and internal rotation, yet no 'reason' for this in the history, then this may simply be an adaptation to the true stressor.

When you desensitise the true stressor, very often this hip range of motion will be restored very quickly without you needing to actually treat it.

Remember, looking at the body and being 'holistic' isn't about treating EVERYTHING; it is simply about working SMARTER and not HARDER. In saying that, if there is a reason for the protective response of a joint, such as pain or trauma, you can use selective tension and various positions to clinically reason which tissues would be a priority to desensitise rather than just throwing everything at it and hoping for the best.

REMEMBER, work SMARTER NOT HARDER.

APPLIED EXAMPLE

A patient is lying supine and you are passively testing their hip flexion. They report a 'pinch' in their groin at 90 degrees with an abrupt end feel. Rather than worry about pathological changes just yet, you would be further strengthening your hypothesis that the passive tissues around the pelvic floor (indirectly via the diaphragm's inability to lengthen also) may not be mobilising.

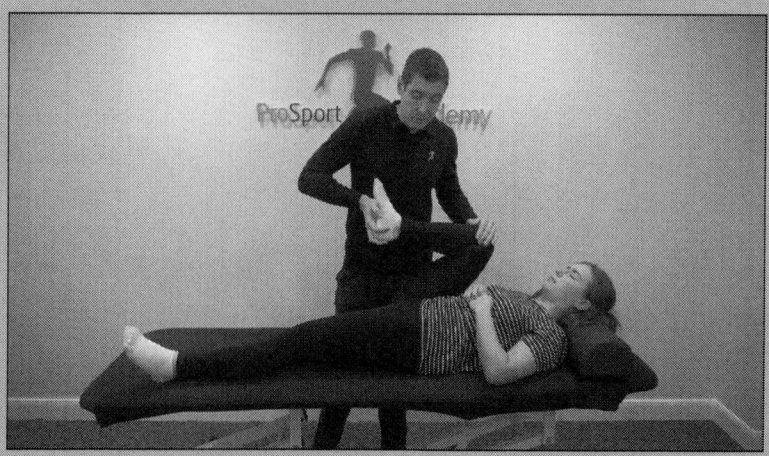

We can then test this by getting the patient to perform a prolonged exhalation and hold their breath at the END of the EXHALATION phase and retest the hip flexion.

If the hip flexion range of motion dramatically improved then this would further strengthen our hypothesis that the pelvic floor may be a main contributor to this back pain or whatever the clinical presentation is.

Other tissues that come to mind if the exhalation did not improve the hip flexion may be the gluteus maximus tissues or adductor magnus, but, again, this would be cross-referenced with the patient's story and the first part of the objective assessment.

IMPORTANT At this point of the assessment you are zoning in on particular tissues to influence positively with your hands-on or hands-off treatment techniques rather than just throwing an elbow in the glutes or 'QL' and 'hoping for the best'.

You have a working hypothesis that some tissues may not be absorbing load efficiently related to adaptations to previous injuries or indirectly via a sensitised respiratory system.

The starting point for the patient in the above applied example may be some respiratory desensitisation techniques designed to mobilise and restore the diaphragm and pelvic floor's ability to move through a full range of motion.

Another great way to clinically reason is to see the difference in hip range of motion supine versus prone.

Certain tissues such as the adductor magnus, for example, will be lengthening in supine while shortening in prone. The difference in gross range of motion between supine and prone would allow us to clinically reason which tissues may be contributing to the reduced range of motion.

If there is a reduced range of motion in supine, for example, then the adductor magnus tissues would be ones we'd be interesting in examining further whereas if the prone range of motion was reduced, then the hip flexor tissues are of more interest as these are lengthening in prone while the adductor magnus tissues are in a shortened position.

Once we go through these interventions, either directly with hands-on treatment, or hands-off with respiratory desensitisation techniques, then the hip range of motion may be restored and we can now focus on the other tissues that are not absorbing load efficiently. We will cover how to do this in the next chapter.

True story: during the initial years I was getting some very good results just using steps 1-3 as my assessment. I was able to help patients become pain-free when jumping off the bed at the end of a session. However, they would come back after a few days or a week later with the pain returning. It was then that **I realised I was missing a step in my system.**

What you know at this point of the assessment is which **tissues have RESPONDED/REACTED/ADAPTED to some perceived threat from the nervous system,** but it **does not tell you WHY these tissues have reacted in this way.**

To find out why, we must add in the final step in the three layer approach.

CHAPTER 8

Step 4 Which directions does the patient not manage perturbatory loads efficiently?

Perturbations that challenge our base of support can happen during all walks of life, especially in high level sporting situations.

These perturbations happen sometimes at such high speeds that the higher centres of the brain don't have time to process this information and so they rely heavily on the peripheral tissues' ability to react and communicate with the spinal cord to maintain equilibrium.

When the foot hits the floor or the hand picks something up, the reality is that the reaction forces will be dealt with throughout the limb and not in one particular direction (sagittal anterior and posterior, frontal medial and lateral, and transverse plane medial and lateral).

If a particular muscle or joint is getting overloaded, for example the adductor, then my first question is why?

Is there another direction that the nervous system is protecting and sending forces in this direction that is now becoming symptomatic?

The motor adaptations to pain or a noxious stimulus are providing interesting insights into how the body can produce the same amount of force through a joint but change the direction of force slightly while also changing the fibres that produce the force (Tucker and Hodges, 2010).

To attempt to find the directions that the body cannot tolerate loading through now, the final part of the 'three-layer approach' is to put a perturbatory load through the tissues and see the response of the nervous system.

However, rather than attempting to isolate a particular muscle, we will apply a pressure no more than 40% of your estimated maximal voluntary contraction through the foot or hand to see how the muscles of the foot, ankle, knee, hip and torso coordinate and manage this perturbatory load in a given direction.

The biggest mistake for therapists who come on my mentorship initially is to think it's a strength test and they apply pressure 100% and try to 'beat' the patient.

All I am interested in here is simply putting a load across a series of joints and checking how the muscles and other tissues within the body deal with this perturbatory load.

Put another way, what you are most interested in is the JOURNEY to the isometric contraction and maintaining voluntary control of the movement after the initial load (or perturbation) is applied to the limb.

The Go-To Therapist is looking for whether a patient uses an immediate high threshold response to a simple task of meeting your pressure at no greater than 40%, or if they can slowly build tension in the muscle proficiently to counteract the load placed on the system by the tester.

This type of assessment approach may give you clues to the muscle's passive and contractile components' ability to generate torque to the task at hand, and to send that force to the tendon while other muscles will be working synergistically to absorb movement errors in order to help the nervous system complete the process.

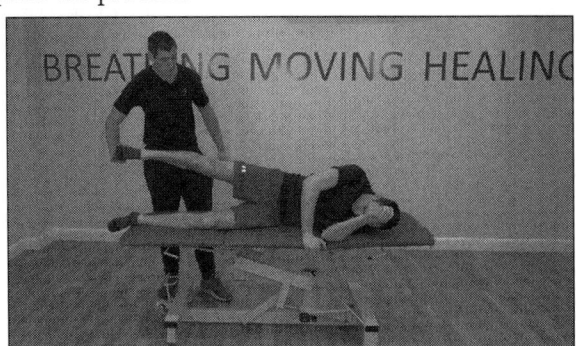

From my observation, a patient that builds tension and brings a MAXIMAL contraction (100% force production) to a task that only requires 40% MVC, for example, is not energy efficient in dealing with the perturbation placed upon the body at this point.

An analogy you may use for patients is that this is like being able to drive a car by only slamming the foot on the accelerator or taking the foot off the accelerator. This strategy is OK short term, and you will get from A to B fast, but there will be potential problems if you have to slow down (deceleration) and turn corners (changing directions).

An inability to bring an efficient motor output to the task is a protective sympathetic response from the nervous system, in my opinion, potentially due to a perceived threat of tolerating load in this direction.

The interesting thing is that this direction will usually be due to a previous injury or an inability of the tissues in this direction to tolerate loading due to stress adaptations, for example.

We would then spend 80% of our time REASSURING the nervous system that it is safe to tolerate loads in this direction. This is done through a step-by-step graded exposure rehab programme which we will cover in the coming chapters.

APPLIED EXAMPLE

If the patient has right-sided groin pain or a recurrent knee pain, yet the same side lateral hip in the posterior lateral direction struggled to generate force efficiently at submaximal levels, then you would still treat the tissues identified in steps 2 and 3 on the right side (20% of your attention) but your rehabilitation focus would be in giving back the body the ability to move with 'thoughtless, fearless movement' biasing the posterior lateral hip through a graded exposure programme (80% of your attention).

It is this approach that has allowed me to help numerous professional and non-sporting patients whose symptoms continued to return. It wasn't until addressing the direction of loading that was inefficient, and restoring movement options and variability of movement so the symptomatic side or direction did not have to perform excessive work that the symptoms fully resolved.

APPLIED EXAMPLE

Another common scenario would be if the patient has right-sided groin pain or a recurrent knee pain yet the OPPOSITE side struggled to generate force efficiently at submaximal levels in a particular direction. You would still treat the tissues identified in steps 2 and 3 on the right side (20% of your attention) but your rehabilitation focus would be in giving back the body the ability to move with 'thoughtless, fearless movement' biasing the OPPOSITE leg through a graded exposure programme (80% of your attention).

This was the case with my professional golfer as mentioned in previous chapters. The key thing here is that there is a reason for the decreased motor output on the opposite leg which you will find in their injury history.

Presently in the Go-To Therapist mentorship I have eight directions in the lower limb, five for the torso and four in the upper limb to build tension and to load these tissues submaximally in the objective assessment.

The hidden benefit of the third layer is that you now have a minimum standard of load tolerance.

My ultimate goal in the first session is to restore the ability to tolerate load through these tissues at around 40% MVC in ALL directions.

When you have helped the patient move pain-free in whatever combination of objective tests you use, the reality is that they can tolerate loading these tissues at that load and that speed. That's it. Just because they can do that does not mean you know they can tolerate the loads required to run, or whatever their goals are. But it gives you something to recheck on the next session so that you can see if they have maintained the progress or regressed again.

This becomes your first Key Performance Indicator (KPI) along with one or two others from the objective assessment.

If the patient leaves with the ability to tolerate load in whatever directions were missing but returns and has lost it again, then I know that either my rehab was too high level or they may have done something between sessions that stressed the system excessively and they have returned to that threatened state.

I would then question the patient about their activities and make sense of why they have lost the ability to tolerate load again in this particular direction.

As we progress the rehab and loading, we will again continue to always recheck these key directions every session as this is our BASELINE tolerance of loading before we progress to increased loading such as standing progressions etc.

This layer is hands down the one which gives me most clarity in terms of where I'll be spending 80% of my attention.

When traditional approaches fail, the problem in the majority of cases is that the clinician has done all the right things on paper with regard to strengthening and loading generally but has just missed the directions that the nervous system needed most. I have seen this even when top-class clinicians were involved.

I personally view this as a coordination problem as opposed to a strength problem as we can change the motor output very quickly with some appropriate hands-on treatment, reassurance and rehab, and witness instant changes in range of motion and other objective tests.

If we bring a strength solution to a coordination problem as most of these failed cases that come to me have had in their previous treatment plans, you will see the problem returning time and time again.

However when we offer reassurance through a step-by-step graded exposure and have the know-how to give the right stimulus at the right time, with the appropriate level of load tolerance, then changes can happen very quickly.

The findings of this layer combined with the other findings and making sense of these with the patient's story would then lead you into effectively explaining your findings to the patient and designing an effective treatment plan.

References mentioned in this chapter:

Tucker KJ, Hodges PW. Changes in motor unit recruitment strategy during pain alters force direction. Eur J Pain. 2010;14(9):932-8.

CHAPTER 9

The 80/20 rule of physical therapy and designing an effective treatment plan

At this point, you now have your 80/20 treatment plan ready to go.

20% of your time (6 minutes in a 30-minute session, 12 minutes in an hour session) is given to desensitising the tissues contributing directly to the pain experience.

This can include your eccentrics, isometrics; whatever you need to do to settle the pain experience.

80% of your time (24 minutes out of 30 or 48 minutes out of a 60-minute session) are given to WHY these tissues have overloaded or become sensitised in the first place.

LOADING AND SPEED OF LOADING

At this point it is important to note that muscles will be able to produce different amounts of force at different speeds as well as different lengths.

Therefore, the speed of the movement and the ability to coordinate this is extremely important to consider when preparing your patient for returning to their activities.

The Go-To Therapist has four key sections that they want their patient to be comfortable with:

- Low Load/Low Speed
- Low Load/Higher Speed
- High Load/Lower Speed
- High Load/High Speed

The Four Different Types of Stimulus Exposed to the Patient on their Return to Meaningful Activities

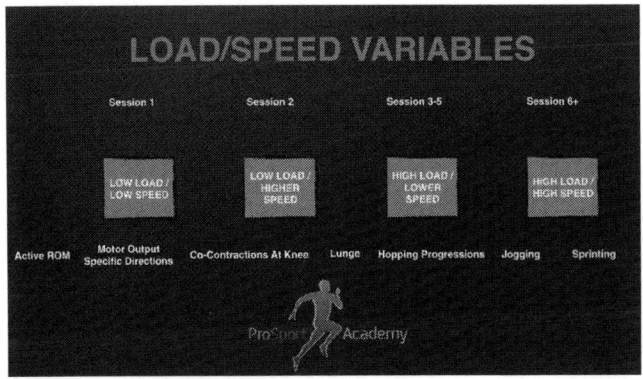

Examples of low load/low speed would be the coordinative testing performed on the bed and low level isometrics.

Examples of low load/high speed would be an 'elastic' lunge in a specific direction.

Examples of high load/low speed would be lifting a kettlebell from the floor in a split stance position with a relaxed back.

Examples of high load/high speed would be hopping progressions, decelerations and sprinting.

You can instantly progress an exercise from low speed to high speed by obviously increasing the speed of the movement; you may then see a completely different movement strategy and this is why it's important to expose your patient to all of these sections in the graded exposure.

A key goal for all our patients is the ability to perform the movements relaxed, both with low and high speed.

It is a far greater challenge to RELAX than it is to TENSE or CONTRACT. Therefore, if a big goal of our rehab plan is to restore coordination and movement efficiency in a specific direction, then performing movements relaxed regardless of load and speed is of utmost importance. This is why I love the phrase 'thoughtless, fearless movement'.

Now let's take you through a clinical scenario of a patient with osteitis pubis who has right-sided groin pain but has a decreased motor output through the same side lateral hip on assessment with a bad previous ATFL injury to the same side ankle.

20% of my time will be focused on desensitising the adductor tissues and 80% on restoring the ability to tolerate load through the peroneal and lateral hip tissues. In the coming chapters, I'll share with you exactly how I'll achieve this.

But first, remember this is just one scenario and you may actually need to look at the opposite leg if your assessment findings take you there.

So the bird's eye view for this treatment plan would be as follows:

Session 1: 20%: Desensitise adductor tissues, reduce pain provocation tests, restore full hip abduction passive length and whatever other reactions were found in the assessment | 80%: Restore motor output through the peroneals and posterior lateral hip at 40% MVC on bed and give isometric equivalent as home exercise programme +/- standing variation.

Session 2: 20%: Recheck hip abduction and pain provocation tests and repeat if required. | 80%: Recheck 40% MVC in each direction on bed, restore if required with hands-on treatment. Progress to standing lower load with higher speed loading.

Session 3: 20%: Asymptomatic with full range or repeat session. | 80% Progress to higher loading with lower speeds.

Session 4: 20%: Asymptomatic. | 80%: Progress to higher loading and higher speed progressions.

Session 5: 20%: Recheck for any adaptations after higher loading and desensitise if required. | 80%: Progress to field deceleration drills, biasing the direction as required.

Session 6: 20%: Recheck for any adaptations after higher loading and desensitise if required. | 80%: Progress to field deceleration drills approx. 90%, biasing the direction as required.

Session 7: 20%: Recheck for any adaptations after higher loading and desensitise if required. | 80%: Progress to final deceleration and acceleration drills, biasing the direction as required at 100% with thoughtless, fearless movement. Plan to discharge with correct graded exposure based movement warm-up in place.

Load/Speed Variables with Progressive Exposure to Load

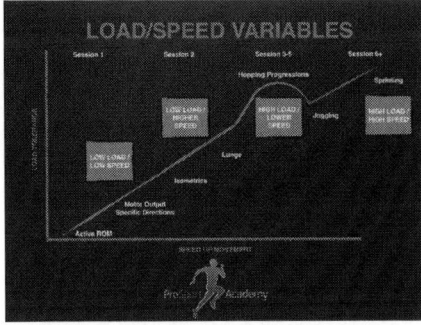

Notice in sessions 1 and 2 how the hands-on treatment was the first step in the graded exposure and by sessions 3–6, there is minimal hands-on treatment, just more reassurance and then it's straight onto the graded exposure.

If you are finding you need to do more and more hands-on treatment as the sessions progress, then I would be concerned that we have not found the true stressors yet and there are considerable adaptations present still.

A big challenge for therapists initially when they come on my mentorship is when to progress a patient or when the patient is ready to run.

The beauty of this way of progressing a patient is we do it through a graded exposure so by the time they've done session 4, we've exposed them to not only similar loads but also greater loads through the tissues that previously had a perceived threat, using techniques that we will cover in the following chapters.

So using some of these simple tweaks, we can bias certain tissues in a controlled environment with ground reaction forces and rates of force development that are actually greater than they need to tolerate when running, for example.

So, for example, if we have a patient that performed our high level hopping progression in session 4 with no reaction in session 5 with regards decreased range of motion, swelling or whatever KPIs we were using, we can be pretty confident now that the patient can tolerate the loading required for running.

You have now logically justified to yourself that the patient has earned the right to progress without second-guessing or making emotional decisions. This is very powerful and will give you amazing confidence and clarity; by this stage your patient will also be feeling very confident.

Progress Loading: Notice how in session 4, the Patient is Exposed to Greater Loads than in Session 5 but in the Controlled Environment of the Clinic.

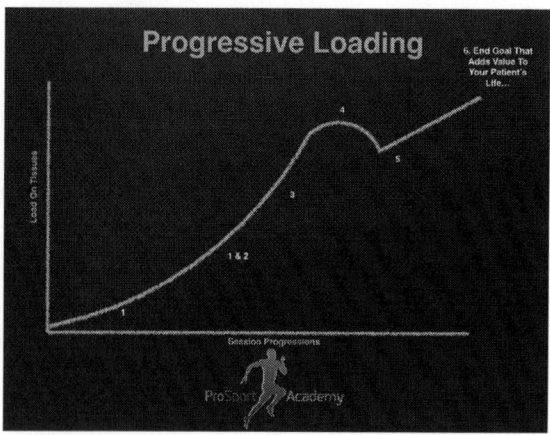

Now let's look at the IMPLEMENTATION of the treatment plan in the real world in the next chapter.

CHAPTER 10

Step 5 Effective explanation for complete patient buy-in and adherence to every exercise

The first step in the treatment process is effective explanation. Pain neuroscience education has become very popular amongst therapists on social media over the last few years.

However, the reality is that when a person is in front of a therapist it is a lot harder to implement than it sounds online. Many therapists are left frustrated by the inability to get the message through to the patient who, after their best efforts, may respond with something like 'so, you're saying it's all in my head?'

The harsh reality is that patients don't really care about pain neuroscience. All patients care about is getting back to what motivated them to come in the first place.

Think about that for a second. A patient is motivated to take action to find a solution for their problem and sought your services for this very reason.

At the end of the day, what a patient really wants to know is what they need to do to get back to what they want to be able to do again.

If you are a non Go-To Therapist and just like the subjective assessment, where you've been focusing on the site of pain and the symptoms, the first words out of your mouth may be the diagnosis.

Patella tendonosis, sciatica, piriformis syndrome...

Once you tell your patient this information, where does their attention go?

What do they tell their partner at home?

What do they then google when they go home, because, let's be honest, they have no idea what that actually means and the second they hear words that are not familiar a subconscious barrier comes up.

The more words in an explanation that a person does not understand, the less confident they will be in gaining understanding and they will give up actively trying.

Think about it...

Recall the last time you read a scientific paper or book that had some words that you didn't understand, or someone tried to explain something and after a few seconds in, you heard two to three words that you were not familiar with and it went way over your head and you naturally started to zone out...

Instead the Go-To Therapist opts for EFFECTIVE EXPLANATION of the actual problem.

There is a big difference between the problem versus the diagnosis.

The diagnosis would be a patella tendonosis but the problem is the hamstring is not working under isometric-like conditions efficiently due to a previous hamstring injury, so the quadriceps are working excessively when decelerating and overloading the patella tendon.

If the person understands the problem, they will then be clear on WHY they are doing an exercise to allow the hamstring an opportunity to work under isometric-like conditions again; from my experience, you will have a far greater chance of patient adherence.

We can still educate the patient on pain neuroscience but rather than use medical words, we use simple terms with the help of diagrams for visual understanding of how the quad muscles are working too hard and putting too much pressure on the knee joint...

...therefore the knee joint is becoming a bit annoyed and sending messages up to the brain that it is doing way too much work because that lazy hamstring is not doing enough work.

If a Person Understands the Problem, then the Next Logical Step is to Find Out the Solution

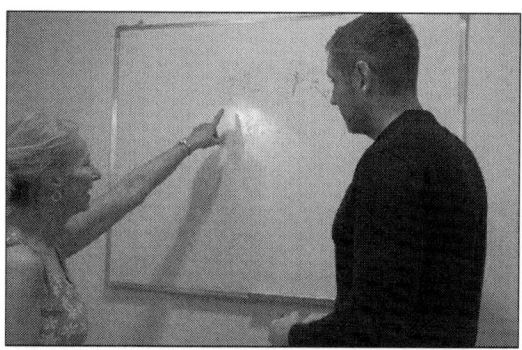

Now what happens is the knee joint actually becomes the GOOD guy and is no longer the victim. This completely changes the patient's perception then of the body part that is in pain, from my experience.

This works brilliantly with back pain patients who think their backs are weak. We then make them realise that their low back is actually doing way too much work because their mid-back or hips, or whatever is the specific problem to the patient, is not doing enough.

The person's perception and relationship with their back then instantly changes and false beliefs and misconceptions are broken effortlessly.

The patient will usually be able to feel the difference in energy expenditure to absorb loads in the directions where there are 'perceived threats' to the system identified in the objective assessment. This will help with the 'buy-in' of the treatment and rehabilitation plan when you are delivering your explanation.

I usually get a lot of 'That makes sense' comments from patients after my explanation, as it is very specific to their story and they can now see how their body has adapted as a result of previous injuries or emotional stressors.

Once the patient understands the problem, they now need to understand the solution.

This is where the Go-To Therapist will explain the step-by-step progressions that need to happen to get that patient back to meaningful activities for them.

The patient will be clear on why they are doing certain exercises but will also understand why they are doing certain things before being able to run, for example.

At the end of the explanation, the patient should be clear on the true problem and what needs to be done to rectify this problem and the step-by-step progressions so that they don't 'try' progress themselves too quickly.

I will then usually give the patient a prognosis of how many sessions this will usually take, based on previous experience, so I can set expectations from the first session.

The final and yet arguably the most important question after informing the patient of how long roughly this will take to resolve is 'Is that what you were expecting?'

This is a great question to avoid having to address any misaligned expectations for the patient that may show up in the second or third session. I'd rather address these issues in the first session along with any objections from the patient in order to leave the path clear to focus completely on getting that patient the meaningful impact.

It may intimidate some therapists to give a prognosis, but professional sports physiotherapists have to do this day in and day out and once you have the confidence and clarity of what has to happen to get the patient the result they want, then this actually works to your advantage.

The other benefit to doing this is it also makes you accountable and focused on the objective of each session.

If you are not where you need to be by session 3, then you may have missed something or haven't found the true stressor. Or you have been ineffective in your treatment stimulus to desensitise what needs to be desensitised.

The great thing is, if your explanation was effective you might actually see the patient's physiology start to change before your eyes.

Physically what is happening, or certainly what I think is happening, is the tone in the diaphragm and pelvic floor relaxes which results in a more slouched position when sitting (which is a good thing by the way!) and the ribcage starts to depress more naturally as the person starts to shift towards the parasympathetic nervous system or 'rest and digest'.

CHAPTER 11

Step 6 Your hands-on treatment is the start of the graded exposure

You are now ready to progress the treatment plan in the form of hands-on treatment. This is the starting point in the person's nervous system's physical load tolerance.

From the objective assessment you will have one to two peripheral tissues that you have identified from steps 2 and 3 to 'desensitise' and reassure the nervous system it is safe for these tissues to absorb load again.

Desensitising these tissues to load will also usually restore the physiological joint range of motion pretty quickly.

We can do this by placing a load via our hands on the areas of the tissues that will need to lengthen during a particular joint movement.

We do this with active movement while reassuring the nervous system further with the help of specific breathing techniques to ensure the patient's autonomic nervous system is in 'rest and digest' at all times.

The direction that we load these tissues and 'reassure' the nervous system will be dependent on the findings of step 4 and the direction that is not tolerating load very well.

For example, let's say our groin pain/osteitis pubis patient had decreased hip flexion and a pinch in the groin mid-range of the 'second third of the physiological joint range of motion'.

Also, our findings were that the gluteus medius tissues have an inability to coordinate with the peroneals and other tissues along that line and work isometrically at a perceived load of around 40% MVC.

We hypothesise the medial direction has been taking more load when decelerating and potentially also pushing off and this has now contributed to groin pain developing on the medial hip area.

This strategy may possibly be due to overloading the medial tissues with ground reaction forces due to an inability to absorb loads through the lateral hip in the posterior lateral direction.

The hands-on treatment intent would be to restore the ability to absorb load through these soft tissues in this area and in the direction of the posterior lateral direction.

This loading locally of the tissues is the starting point of the graded exposure in restoring the ability to tolerate load in the particular direction identified. This will then be progressed straight away with step 7.

It is important to note that the intention of the hands-on treatment approach is not to break up scar tissue or anything like that but to simply REASSURE the nervous system it is safe to tolerate load in the direction you've identified in the assessment.

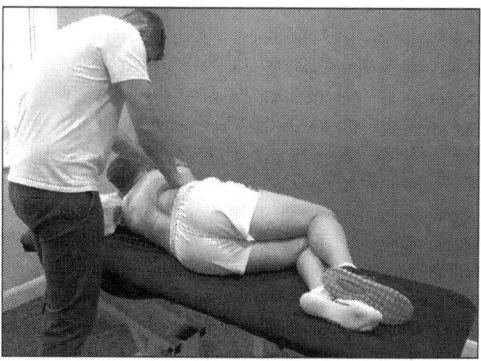

A better term may be the ability to tolerate tension. We want these tissues to tolerate tension which is important for movement efficiency and coordination because when these tissues tension or lengthen their receptors will be stimulated, giving important sensory information to the spinal cord and higher centres.

A higher level strategy for the Go-To Therapist is to simply restore full physiological joint range of motion and the ability to tolerate load through these tissues in every direction. We give the nervous system access to as close to full sensory information as possible and then leave it to figure out the rest.

The biggest mistake I see therapists make with hands-on treatment is to be too compressive. Compressing tissues and then asking them to lengthen while keeping them compressed will usually put too much tension on some parts of the tissue and not enough on other parts. From my experience, this will result in the patient going into 'fight or flight' as can be witnessed with their breathing strategies and the tension in their whole body.

It is important to point out also that the exact mechanism of why this works is still unclear. I am very comfortable in 'not' knowing the exact mechanism and resisting the urge to make up 'far-fetched' explanations to the patient. Remember at all times, WE are the GUIDE and NOT the HERO in this story. The patient is the HERO.

Therefore my explanation is a very simple one that informs the patient that I am just helping them to tolerate some loading going through these tissues again and helping them update their nervous system's belief that it is now safe to use these tissues again.

The actual hands-on strategy should look something like this:

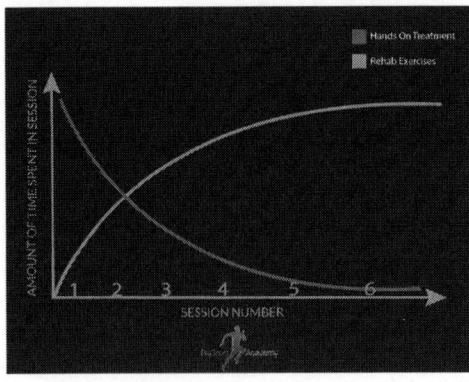

The Go-To Therapist Will Actually Do Less Hands-on Treatment and More Movement-based Rehab as the Sessions Progress

The first session or two is when the majority of hands-on treatment takes place and then, as we progress through the treatment plan, the majority of time is taken up coaching and reassuring the patient in the movements that there are still 'perceived threats' present or where further graded exposure in the loading plan is still needed.

Towards sessions 4 or 5 there should actually be very little, if any, hands-on treatment taking place. A quick reassessment of the objective assessment and coordination testing and you should be good to go with the next progressions.

If the patient has slightly reduced physiological joint range of motion, then it is OK to help them restore this quickly with hands-on if you wish, although the graded exposure warm-up will usually get this back anyway.

The key component to the hands-on treatment desensitisation for me is the clinical reasoning of WHY you are needing to desensitise these tissues in the first place. If these tissues relate to the injury history or have meaning for the patient's story, then that is great. If they don't and it is simply a reaction, then I am slow to desensitise tissues just for the sake of it and would rather step back and think on a higher level of WHY these tissues have reacted like this in the first place.

The final thing I want to warn you about also is to respect the need for a graded exposure plan.

The novel stimulus applied by your hands with your first treatment session will usually create some kind of nervous system response/adaptation anyway and this can be a tripwire for therapists and patients where the patient leaves the session feeling great but then the pain comes back again shortly after.

The trap some therapists can fall into then is to repeat the same hands-on treatment process. What they commonly find is that in the second session, there is some relief in symptoms but it is not as great as in the first session, which can be puzzling for both the therapist and the patient. However, the problem, in my opinion, is that this hands-on treatment is a little bit less novel now and so the reaction for the nervous system is not as great.

Therefore this is why I believe you truly need to have that step-by-step graded exposure plan in place to keep the gains between sessions, to ensure the pain or loss in range of motion does not return and to get the patient capable of tolerating these loads at both high loads and high speeds, specific to their needs to be able to enjoy their life.

Let's now look in the next chapter at what the Go-To Therapist will do after applying the hands-on treatment to the patient.

CHAPTER 12

Step 7 Restoring the ability to build tension and work synergistically

So far you have reassured the patient's nervous system locally that it is safe to tolerate load at some starting point level of load tolerance in this particular direction. We now want to further expose these tissues to absorbing force and dealing with it effectively in partnership with its muscle synergies, and to distribute this load through the limb and not excessively in one particular place.

Such an example of this may be absorbing excessive load in the hamstrings, whereby the hamstrings cramp when performing a single leg bridge for example. I would very much view this as a protective response from the nervous system.

The use of a submaximal isometric exercise is the next logical progression to exposing these tissues to load, an opportunity to overcome muscle slack while also potentially undoing any fascicle length changes within the local tissues.

Most importantly this will also help restore the nervous system's ability to generate a force along these tissues, dampen it with the tendons and spread it throughout the body more efficiently.

The use of an isometric is to simply continue to expose the tissues to load but give an opportunity/environment for the nervous system to coordinate this process while in a state of 'rest and digest'.

The Go-To Therapist will achieve this by integrating respiratory desensitisation techniques here to ensure the person is in 'rest and digest' while restoring the ability to generate tension at submaximal levels. This exercise is not a max strength isometric but rather a submaximal and gradual build in pressure which will bring the patient's conscious awareness back to these body parts and restore control at submaximal levels.

The critical point here, however, is that the loading of these tissues is in the direction that we have identified from step 4 and is the next natural progression of loading from step 6.

Although some therapists believe exercises do not need to be specific and the benefits are non-specific, from my experience the ability to load certain parts of tissues can massively accelerate the patient's confidence and movement capabilities whereas just doing the isometrics do not achieve this.

An example of this would be seen in the image below. We can see here two different isometric exercises for the lateral hip, where one would be targeting the hip tissues in the frontal plane while the other would be targeting the transverse plane loading of the hip.

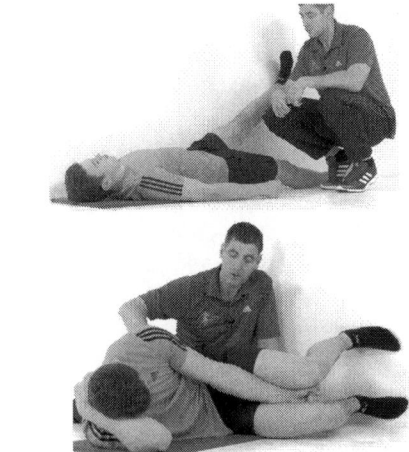

The exercise choice you would use would be dependent on the assessment findings, specifically from step 4.

Whenever there is an opportunity to load a tissue isometrically, I like to make use of the ability of the nervous system to coordinate this loading with muscle synergies and antagonists by utilising the hand or foot also.

Using these joints will also help coordinate the tissues that will usually be working together in real life and will add more problems and meaning for the nervous system to figure out, in my opinion.

For the upper limb, the Go-To Therapist would send the load through the fingers and wrist first in a certain direction to get the cuff and trapezius muscles, for example, working in coordination with the hand, wrist and elbow joints.

For the torso, the Go-To Therapist would spread the load through both the hands and feet, as required, in the given directions.

This chapter is not long as we do not need to complicate this process. The aim of step 7 is to simply continue to give the tissues an opportunity to tolerate load in a 'safe' environment, ideally while coordinating with the other joints in the limb.

And if you actually think about it, just like the step 4 testing, it is the journey to the isometric contraction that is more important than the isometric contraction itself.

This step would happen immediately after step 6's hands-on treatment for an area and would utilise usually about a loading for 6-8 breaths for about 6 seconds each rep.

CHAPTER 13

Step 8 Graded exposure to meaningful movements

The next step straight after the isometrics in step 7 is to get the patient straight up onto their feet and to move in meaningful ways that we have identified from step 1 in understanding the person's story and what really adds value to their life.

It is important to start the process straight away of getting the patient back on track towards that end goal. We can modify these meaningful movements by using low loads and low speeds to start with until the patient's confidence starts to grow.

With the meaningful movements, we again want the body to 'self-organise' and figure out the movement strategy subconsciously as has to happen in the majority of tasks in the real world rather than focusing on internal cues such as 'squeeze your glutes' or 'pull your belly button in' etc.

To implement this in the real world, the Go-To Therapist will focus the patient's attention on the outcome of the task rather than specific internal cues, to replicate how movement tasks are executed in the real world.

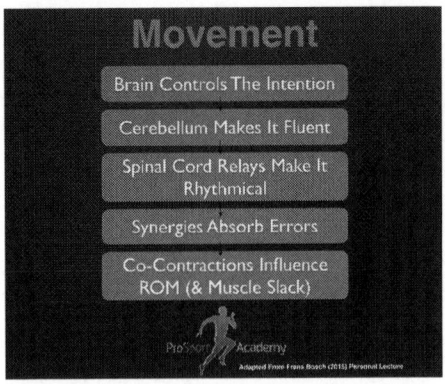

Movement, Adapted from Frans Bosch Lecture to the Go-To Therapist Mentorship Group, 2015.

You will give the person a clear focus and use the outcome of the task to challenge their base of support to provide the body with the ability to self-organise on numerous levels while under perturbatory loads.

Managing unexpected perturbatory loads is a key part of being successful in both sport and life and we need to provide the patient an opportunity to be exposed to these loads and let their nervous system figure it all out.

Now this is not to say we just put them in a position and give them a nudge and say 'hey, figure this out yourself!'; this part is arguably the piece that therapists fall down on most commonly. There really is an art to progressing a patient without irritating them or causing negative reactions within their system.

The four variables of low load, low speed and high load, high speed and combinations of these become extremely valuable and important to the therapist during the graded exposure process.

So now let's get back to our groin pain patient and recap their treatment intervention so far.

The patient has had an effective explanation of the true problem (why the groin area is overloading) and the solution (get the posterior lateral hip to share the workload) and understands that the adductor muscles are not the bad guys after all but are just grumpy and letting the patient know they are doing too much work.

They then received some hands-on loading to the lateral hip as the first step in getting the nervous system confident in tolerating load in this direction which in total probably took no more than two minutes.

The therapist uses a key performance indicator such as gross range of motion or motor output in that direction (like the step 4 coordination assessment) to gauge how effective the hands-on treatment intervention was.

Immediately after the hands-on treatment, the patient will perform 6–8 reps of an isometric exercise that gives the nervous system an ability to continue to tolerate load in the direction it received from the hands-on treatment but which now includes the muscle synergists and antagonists to coordinate with the other joints in the limb. They will also be using respiratory desensitisation techniques to further bring the nervous system into 'rest and digest' while tolerating loads that previously were associated with having a 'perceived threat'.

Now we get the patient straight up to their feet after performing six to eight reps of the exercise chosen in the previous chapter for the next progression. The total physical treatment/intervention time to date is around four minutes.

As you can see in the example on the next page, the reach of the left hand is now driving the pelvis outside the base of support which will cause pre-reflexive and reflexive-like reactions at the local tissues while also showing the nervous system it is safe to load the lateral hip tissues with greater loads placed upon the body.

In this movement, the nervous system has no other option but to decelerate the body weight with the lateral hip tissues.

This is a simple way to get a load through certain tissues if we understand the reactions that happen through the body with certain movements. A physical therapist in the U.S called Gary Gray first coined the term 'chain reaction' to describe this.

The Go-To Therapist will, however, understand which directions are priorities for the patient at each loading phase through the assessment which will give greater clarity and save time in giving the appropriate stimulus rather than using multiple exercises in the session.

The Go-To Therapist once again appreciates the four variables and understands how and when to progress the patient with low load, high load, low speed and high speed variations.

This thought process can be used with any injury.

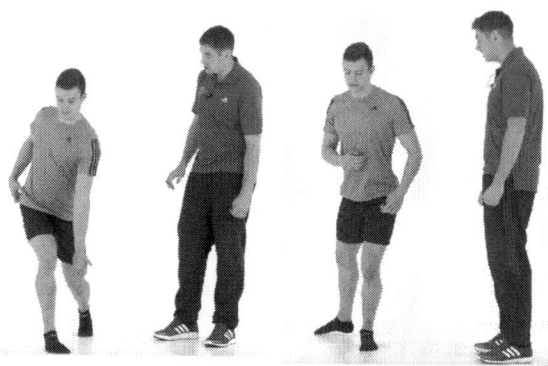

As you can see here with the other image on the right, if we used this kind of loading it would stress the tissues on the medial side of the hip.

So, for example, in the 2017 Rugby League World Cup, I was using the movement on the left with an MCL injury in week one where we wanted to load the injured tissues a little, but the majority of force was absorbed through the lateral tissues.

In the following week when we wanted to increase load through the MCL tissues to decrease perceived threats and force the medial hamstrings to absorb more load as the tissue healing times are more appropriate, we used the image on the right.

The other great benefit of operating like this is that it is also the start of our exposure to change of direction, so by the time we need the patient to twist and turn at high speeds, the exact same tissues have been experiencing appropriate loads going through them and the higher centres are not perceiving these as threats.

It is this ART of graded exposure where there is clarity in how every exercise movement builds onto the next until it all comes together that I truly believe can cut days and weeks off potential return to play times.

So while some therapists in session 1 are focusing on the site of pain and massaging the area etc., the Go-To Therapist is already focusing and working on a graded exposure for the change of direction component of the return to play.

By the time I get patients back to running (if that's where we need to get the patient back to), the work done in sessions 1 and 2 gives a great foundation and the patient will usually fly when progressing into the graded exposure running progressions.

So now back to our groin pain patient.

The exercise progression may finish session 1 and so their rehab programme between sessions is simply the isometric variation from the previous chapter and the standing progression from this chapter.

Ideally when leaving after session 1, the patient has restored full physiological joint range of motion and can tolerate loading in each of the eight directions for the lower limb or the four directions for the upper limb etc.

So in the groin pain patient's example, we would ideally want to have restored full hip flexion and the motor output at 40% MVC in all eight directions of both limbs.

When the patient returns for session 2, the Go-To Therapist will recheck the key performance indicators such as the one to two objective assessment movements and also the direction of force testing from step 4.

Ideally when the patient returns they will still be able to display a good motor output in all eight directions. This would be a great sign that they have maintained the tolerance load between sessions and are ready to further progress in the graded exposure ladder.

If the patient came in and they were back to how they were pre-treatment in session 1, there would then be a conversation mapping out step-by-step what they did between when they left after session 1 and now, to find out exactly why they have regressed again.

Usually if they have regressed it can be due to the exercises being too high load for this point (which is rare); the patient doing the exercises incorrectly or not following instructions; or the patient feeling a bit better and pushing ahead with activities that are too high level, in which case we would need to review the effective explanation section again as we did not do a good enough job communicating the plan.

For the sake of our groin pain patient, we are going to assume that you have done a great job with your effective explanation and with your hands-on treatment and rehab choices for session 1 and the KPIs you are working with are going to plan. When your patient next comes in, you need to progress them onto the next step of the graded exposure plan.

CHAPTER 14

Step 9 Progressively load the movement and outcomes

When the patient returns, we would make sure the KPIs are all going in the right direction including the patient's symptoms. The KPIs for this patient would be their hip flexion passive assessment and also their motor output in the direction of the posterolateral hip. The other KPI you might be interested in would be the adductor squeeze scores which may have been painful and/or weak.

At this point in the rehab, sessions 2-3, the patient will usually be feeling pretty good and asking when they can run again, for example. The problem is, up to this point I have absolutely NO IDEA if they can tolerate higher ground reaction forces, especially in the directions we've identified in step 4.

The big question is whether with these higher demands, they will be able to tolerate loads through these paths or go back to old movement habits and load excessively in the areas where the symptoms were first experienced.

It is also worth noting that you have only stressed these tissues to date at low loads and low speeds.

To avoid guessing if the patient is ready to run, step 9 is all about progressively loading the tissue identified and increasing the demands on the patient's nervous system through a graded exposure at higher loads and higher speeds of movement.

It is very common for the patient to be looking really good at lower speeds and loads but once we speed the movement up, they revert back to older movement habits.

Remember: A NEW LEVEL OF LOADING, A NEW PROBLEM FOR THE NERVOUS SYSTEM TO FIGURE OUT.

We can expose the patient's nervous system to these loads by increasing the speed of movements or by other means via single leg loading which will continue to challenge the base of support further.

You can also further threaten the nervous system by repeating the single leg variation but on a box or height.

Think about walking along a two by four plank of wood on the floor and then repeating this on a small height in the playground versus the same plank but between two skyscraper buildings.

The height variable further increases the perceived threat to the nervous system and hence the patient will tend to go towards 'fight or flight', change their breathing strategy and usually decrease their movement variability. We can use this knowledge to our advantage when prescribing rehab exercise progressions in the real world.

You will be watching the patient's reactions closely to understand if he/she is ready to progress further or needs to regress. You can access a free bonus training on this using the link below:

FOR FREE PROGRESSIONS AND REGRESSIONS TRAINING VISIT

www.thegotophysiobook.com/resources

The progressions for the groin pain patient in sessions 2 and 3 may start with a lunge movement with the perturbatory load applied as the foot hits the floor at higher speeds and then progress to a single leg variation in session 3 as shown in the image on the following page.

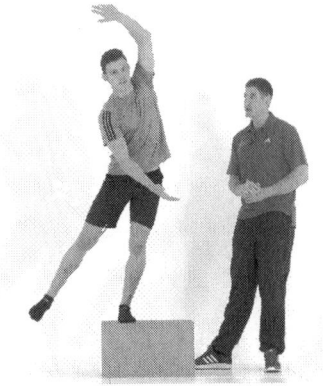

As you can see by the reach of the arm, we can continue to load the lateral hip tissues effortlessly (the left side in this image) with more challenges for the nervous system to overcome, such as the box height, to name but one.

If the patient is OK with these loads, and has no negative reactions to the KPIs, then it is time to progress to step 9.

It is worth noting that as you progress your patient to higher loads, new problems may become evident, specific to their story and injury history that did not flag up on your basic assessment.

These loading exercises are also used as assessments now and it is worth putting these levels of load across all directions for the limb quickly in the session to screen for any 'energy inefficiencies' at certain loads or speeds of movement that our basic lower level assessments in session 1 and 2 may have missed.

Remember, A NEW LEVEL OF LOADING, A NEW PROBLEM FOR THE NERVOUS SYSTEM TO FIGURE OUT and this is why at each level going forwards, we will check all planes of movement for any 'energy inefficiencies'.

These inefficiencies will usually be related to the person's story and may require some hands-on treatment to help desensitise further and a week spent on tolerating loads at this level and speed, before progressing to higher loads and speeds in the graded exposure plan.

If all is well and you've cleared any potential problem areas, then you are good to progress to step 10 in the next chapter.

CHAPTER 15

Step 10 How to know EXACTLY WHEN the patient is ready to return to running or other high load activities

In my experience, this step is the most commonly omitted step in the majority of rehab programmes that have failed traditional approaches.

To have complete confidence that the patient is ready to return to running or other high loading and high speed activities, the Go-To Therapist needs to be able to justify this logically and without emotion playing a part.

I see so many therapists making these decisions emotionally and wanting to 'please' the patient or almost getting clues from the patient rather than remaining the authority and guiding the patient.

In order to justify this logically, the Go-To Therapist needs to make sure that there is no doubt the patient can tolerate even higher levels of ground reaction forces through the direction that was identified as having a 'perceived threat' present in the initial assessment and/or other directions that they picked up during the higher levels of loading.

You can see by the progressive loading plan on the next page that session 4's exposure to load for our groin pain patient will actually be greater than what the patient will actually be tolerating in session 5 when they go back for their first running session.

Therefore, in theory, if they can come through session 4 without any reaction from the nervous system in the form of pain, swelling, range of motion restrictions, or whatever other KPIs you are using, you can be pretty confident the patient will be able to tolerate the loading in the next session.

Progressive Loading Progressions

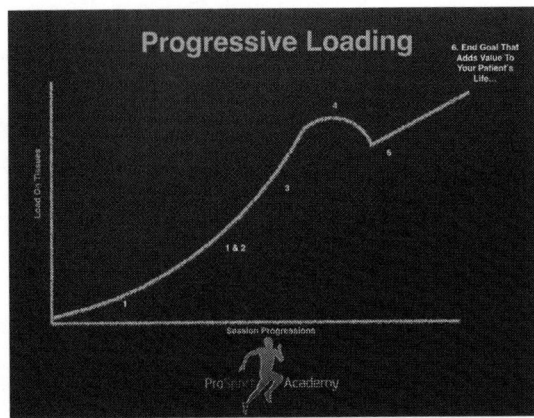

We do this by going through a specific step-by-step set of hopping progressions I've used successfully over the last ten years working in professional sport.

As you can see from the chart on the next page, taken from the Scarfe et al (2011) paper, the ground reaction forces for a hop are actually greater than jogging, which logically makes sense.

When we use our knowledge about different reactions that happen to the body to bias certain directions with even more load, we can then further expose certain 'directions' with more load than others, like we have done in the previous 3-4 sessions with the patient.

Therefore, logically then, if there are no reactions from the hopping progressions and the groin pain patient is able to do these movements with 'thoughtless, fearless movement' in the specific planes and directions that they previously struggled with, then the next progression would be to start running.

Ground Reaction Forces and Rate of Force Development for Various Movements

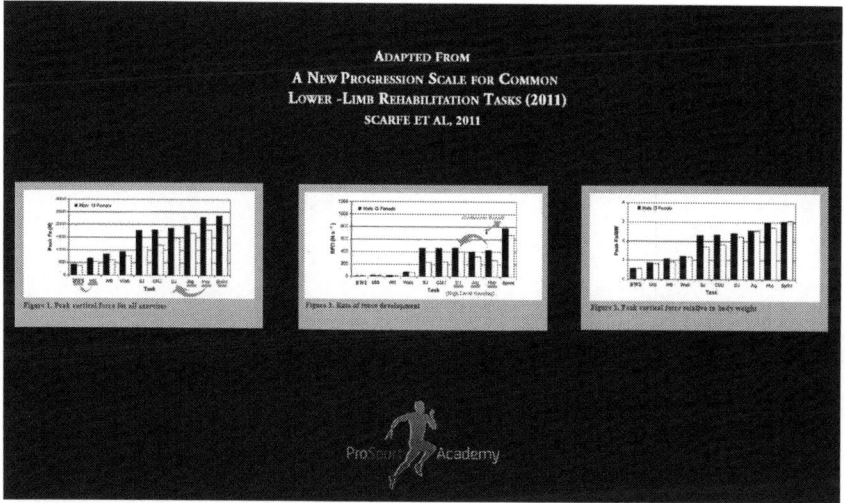

Now, before we go ahead with the running progressions, there are some limitations to relying on hopping as a 'fail safe' way to put load on the tissues as you can see above in the image.

There is quite a gap in the rate of force development between hopping and sprinting, which would be our final session in the graded exposure programme. To combat this problem, the hopping progressions need to take this into consideration with the progressions used. Therefore I have had to come up with some custom variations of traditional hopping to increase both the rate of force development and the ground reaction forces, to be certain the patient can tolerate these loads before allowing them to sprint in the final running progressions.

Working this way allows me to have complete clarity and confidence that I have logically justified the progressions and the patient is indeed ready to return running.

So, for example, with our groin pain patient, the first level of hopping progression would be leaping from one leg and landing on the other.

As you can see in the image below, we asked the athlete to finish the movement with a reach across their body just as they land.

To self-organise and stabilise their centre of gravity between the base of support, the pelvis will again need to travel laterally, and the lateral hip tissues will be forced to decelerate the bodyweight.

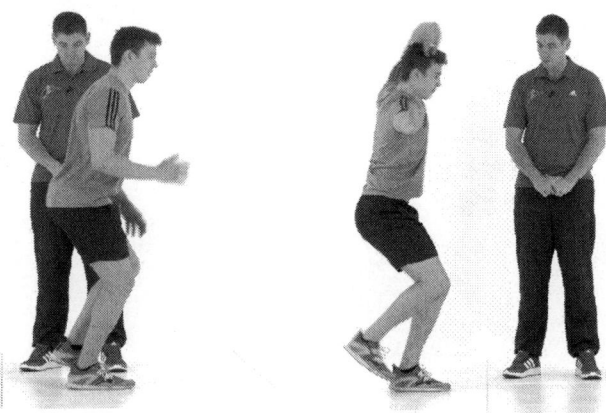

If we go through the next higher level hopping progressions and there are no adverse reactions from the nervous system (such as reduced motor outputs upon retesting, reduced range of motion, swelling, or whatever markers you are using), then I am very confident this groin pain patient is ready to start running.

When the patient is back running in the next step, the whole limb will be contributing without having to bias a particular direction like we have been doing, so in actual fact there will be even less load on the tissues that had the original 'threat response'.

This is what gives me complete confidence because we know the patient can tolerate even higher forces than the ground reaction forces they will need to endure when running.

The hopping progressions can all be progressed in the same session if the patient is ready to do so – it is completely down to the person in front of you. I would then leave them with the highest loading progressions with the highest rate of force development for a week, or a day or so, if in a pro sport setting, and reassess for any negative reactions. If all is good, then we progress the patient to 11.

It is worth mentioning again that at this point in the treatment plan I quickly screen all planes and directions of loading for any 'energy inefficiencies' that did not show up until this level and speed of loading.

It is not uncommon to see a big discrepancy in force absorption or force production at these high levels that were not picked up on with the previous levels of load.

If there are 'energy inefficiencies' present, especially in the highest hopping progressions for an elite athlete, then this may not set us back in terms of prognosis for return to play but rather offer insight into what the athlete needs to be focusing on when they return to team training. Also, this work may actually be integrated into their strength and conditioning programme to ensure they build resilience which we will talk about in more detail in step 12.

The final point to mention in this chapter is that you may not have to take all your patients through the high level hopping progressions that are mentioned in this chapter. If you have a patient that wants to just get back to lifting their kids or grandkids, then this step's level of loading may in fact be external weight such as kettlebells or barbells etc where we have some control of the quantity of loading.

However, I would take the majority of my lower limb patients certainly through the leaping progressions as a minimum as the majority of people need to be able to run for a bus some day or run after their kids so I like them to be able to tolerate this level of loading before moving onto the more resilience-based focus of the graded exposure programme.

With that said, let's now move on to the running progressions for our groin pain patient in the next chapter.

CHAPTER 16
Step 11 Return to running acceleration and deceleration progressions

From here, step 11 is very straightforward if you have progressed the athlete or patient appropriately to date.

The return to running progressions is mostly the same continuation of exposure to load but obviously at higher speeds now.

The first running session aim is to get up to 70% of the max speed in both force production and force absorption.

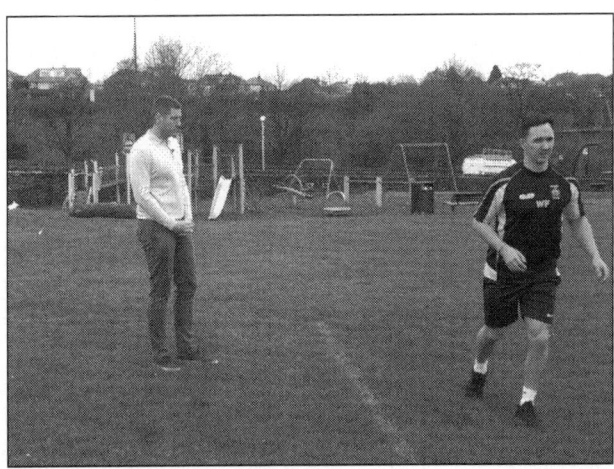

The Go-To Therapist will use a tempo running protocol of increasing intensity over the course of three-plus sessions, but, if done right and with medium-term injuries, should not need much more than three running sessions, with the exception of course in scenarios where the athlete has deconditioned such as ACL injuries.

The Go-To Therapist's running sessions will also be including frontal and transverse plane loading for force absorption needs in particular. This again is an opportunity to screen for any 'energy inefficiences' that we may not have picked up previously with different loads and speeds of movement.

The directions of loading can be biased further, just like you have done the whole way through the graded exposure plan, by using the hands, for example, to further challenge the body's base of support if needed.

The first session's aim is to hit 70% max speed on the final two tempo runs and also hit 70% deceleration in the sagittal, frontal and transverse planes.

The nice advantage of not hitting more than 70% in the first session is that the athlete will usually be OK to run again the next day, if in the professional or semi-professional setting. You will continue to monitor closely as always for any negative reactions to your KPIs the following day before allowing to progress.

By session 2, the aim is to progress to 90% max speed by the final two tempo runs and decelerations in all three planes of motion. The same principles apply of monitoring for any negative reactions or 'energy inefficiencies' throughout and the following day.

I personally like the athlete or patient to have a rest day the following day if they have hit 90% in this session on their final few runs.

In the final running session, the aim would be to hit 100% top end speed and intent with decelerations in three planes of motion along with some unpredictability built into the session, especially during the change of direction loadings. The athlete or patient needs to be able to move with complete 'thoughtless, fearless movement' in all directions and planes of movement in this session before being discharged or allowed to return to training.

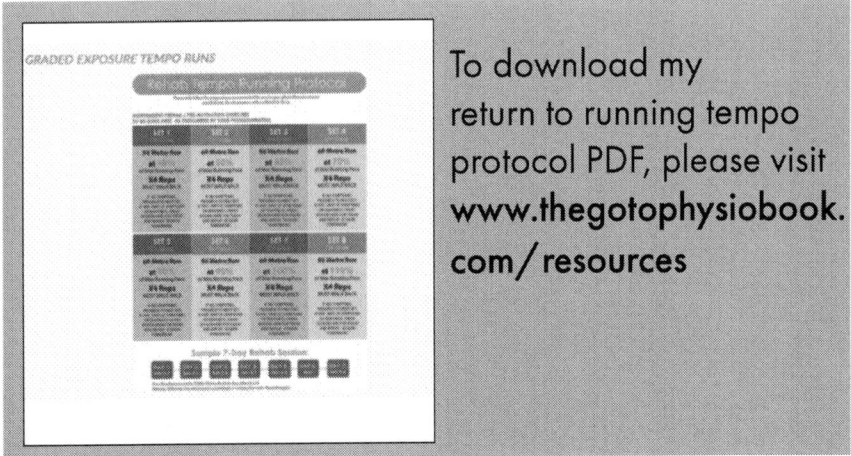

To download my return to running tempo protocol PDF, please visit **www.thegotophysiobook. com/resources**

If the person is preparing for a contact sport then the contact integration will also be done over the three sessions in a graded exposure with a predictable to unpredictable progressive manner.

If you are in private practice, then you may not be able to work on the tempo runs in the clinic for obvious reasons. However, to do an effective deceleration programme in three planes of motion, this can be executed in a ten-square-foot treatment room easily for the first couple of sessions and the patient can perform their tempo runs on a field independently with clear instructions to follow. You do not need to have a lot of space for effective deceleration work to really challenge the speed and load placed on the patient's nervous system.

Another nice benefit of this progressive step-by-step manner is that your patient's warm-up for these running sessions is simply the exercises they have been performing over the past few sessions to get that graded exposure to load before the running takes place. The sets can essentially be reduced to one to two sets and the reps reduced to suit the athlete's needs also.

You may also choose to integrate additional general mobility drills into the warm-up if required. The patient is so familiar with the cueing of the exercises plus the ability to now decelerate efficiently, that the running sessions, from my experience, tend to go very smoothly, especially if we have not missed any 'energy inefficiencies' in the preceding sessions.

Other therapists are not necessarily wrong in their approach to run athletes as soon as possible, but I am personally in no rush to run the athlete as I prefer to build a solid foundation and decrease the risk of developing further motor adaptations while pain or nervous system adaptations are still present. Although this may look like it will take my athletes longer to get back, I actually find the opposite as from day 1 post injury, for this groin pain patient, I am working on his/her graded exposure to change of direction and force production for acceleration and top end speed, specific to his/her needs.

Although I am in no rush to run my athlete, I will spend a lot more time on step 10 and the hopping progressions, so when the patient returns to running, they are more than capable of managing the ground reaction forces and perturbatory forces at said rate of force development.

It is imperative, in my opinion, that the patient is exposed to the loads and speeds of movement that they will be exposed to in training or games, before returning to these. I see so many athletes returning to training when they've hit 80% max speed, for example, without actually hitting the top speeds and then they have protective responses when they do open up or move at a speed that they had not been exposed to previously in the rehab process. It is a risky way of working, and not one the Go-To Therapist would utilise to ensure consistently long-lasting results.

Once the patient or athlete returns to the training environment, it is also very important that they continue with the bespoke graded exposure warm-up prior to taking part in the team warm-up, especially for the first three to six sessions.

Keeping it simple, you want to give them a graded exposure to the load and speeds they will need to tolerate in the training session so ideally the first time they are exposed to these loads won't be in the training session. While it is impossible to ensure this every session, it can give you good direction for pre-training movement prep and 'injury prevention programmes'.

The patient's KPIs will also be monitored pre-training, if possible in the professional setting, depending on equipment requirements. For our groin pain patient, the adductor squeeze and posterolateral hip force production may be monitored in the professional environment closely pre-training. For the weekend warrior, a simple 'perception' of how their adductor squeeze feels while pushing their knees into their hand may suffice in getting a gauge of how much pre-training graded exposure may be needed. For something like an ankle injury we can teach the non-sporting patient to use a ruler to measure their knee to wall lunge test for gross ankle range of motion as a more straightforward method.

In regards to getting the ideal pre-training warm-up, I believe this is down to an athlete's perception and personal feel but certainly it makes sense to me to include a graded exposure to load and speed of movement to logically justify eliminating the chances of 'perceived threats' kicking in.

Once the patient is back successfully achieving the tasks that add value to their lives, then it is time to turn our attention to building some resilience in these tasks, especially under times of high stress.

CHAPTER 17

Step 12 Build resilience under external loads and increased stress

The final step in the Go-To Therapist method is to utilise the ability to generate tension in these muscles in all directions and build strength.

In this stage, you will ensure your patient can tolerate the load and still move with good movement variability and weight distribution through the hand or foot.

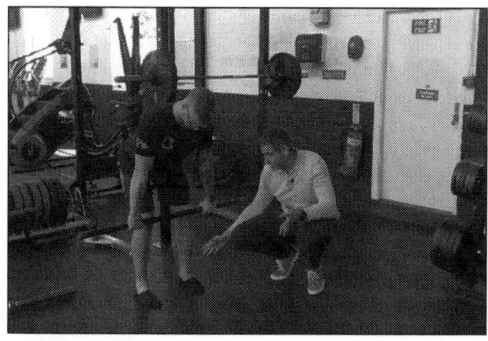

I don't agree with the notion that just getting people strong is enough. I have worked for ten-plus years with strong athletes that were in pain.

Therefore, this step happens after the nervous system is happy to generate tension in all directions. We can still achieve a task of heavy deadlifting weights but the adductor magnus, for example, may be creating additional torque if the lateral hip tissues are still not proficient and are perceived as a threat.

So, just like every other step in this process, the Go-To Therapist's patients earn the right to be at this stage at the appropriate time. The athlete/patient will get even stronger when he/she has plenty of movement options and the actual ability to produce force through as many motor units as possible.

At this stage, from my experience, you will see a significant increase in strength and power capabilities once the right has been earned to be at this level.

The patient does not necessarily need to wait until progressing to step 12 to start additional loading and, indeed, depending on the patient's needs, will actually start external loading in step 8 if that is what is needed, specific to that patient.

This step is more concerned with building general resilience to various loads placed on the body both mentally and physically.

The Go-To Therapist will achieve good movement variability and physical resilience by ensuring there is good weight distribution through the whole foot and hand when lifting external loads.

One of the biggest mistakes I see being made by strength and conditioning coaches in this day and age is an obsession with everything having to be pushed through the heels.

The athlete starts on the heels and finishes on the heels. This is one sure way to ensure decreased movement variability, coordination and an inability to react to perturbatory loads from different angles.

The Go-To Therapist will logically think about it and look at Olympic weightlifters and the gait cycle, and see that during times of hip extension, when we need good coordination to manage big loads, we need the weight distribution to be going towards the midfoot and forefoot, not stuck on the heels.

I personally believe this cue to push through the heels is ingrained and reinforces poor coordination patterns, making athletes less efficient in the long run. The Go-To Therapist wants their patients to be able to have good movement variability and manage their weight as it travels towards the heel when the hip flexes and travels towards the mid- to forefoot when the hip extends.

Another big goal for the Go-To Therapist is to help build mental resilience for the patient. It is, in my opinion, important to expose the patient to environments or situations that will bring them into the sympathetic nervous system dominance.

This is inevitable in everyday life.

What is most important for the patient is to be able to get back out of sympathetic dominance again and into the parasympathetic or 'rest and digest' system.

These scenarios can be stressful situations or environments such as at home or work, or at training for the athlete. We need the patient to be able to utilise their sympathetic nervous system but then when the stressor is removed, revert back into their parasympathetic nervous system and recover and regenerate.

For example, this type of resilience training would be appropriate for those patients with persistent back pain before going to sleep to ensure they are actually in rest and digest before sleeping and also first thing in the morning when waking.

Integrating this type of intervention can have massive effects on overall mood, mindset and quality of life from my personal observation with patients. I'm sure you too have witnessed the power of a good night's sleep on mood, movement and mindset.

And that is the complete step-by-step system that I've been using successfully over the last few years with athletes or private practice patients who come to me, who have on paper done everything 'right' and have been under the care of some top-class physios but may just have skipped a step or two in their plan.

The most overlooked or 'missed' step in the 12-step method is step 1 – not understanding the patient's story thoroughly – which makes it almost impossible to make sense of the objective assessment and consequent steps thereafter.

Then, after this, I believe it would be step 4 and not understanding WHY the REACTIONS and SYMPTOMS have happened in the first place. So while most therapists are focusing their time on the symptoms, it only accounts for 20% of the Go-To Therapist's time and 80% of their time is spent focusing on the tissues that are not doing enough in the first place that caused these reactions.

Once you have identified these directions of force, then it will just be slight tweaks in your exercises to stimulate specific directions of loading that are currently being avoided. You will usually notice quick changes and then it is just a case of giving the patient the right stimulus at the right time in the graded exposure programme.

At all times, ensure your patient has clarity on the problem and the solution (graded exposure rehab programme) which is meaningful to their situation. The outcomes will add value to their life and you will never have a problem with patient motivation, adherence or a patient dropping off.

Remember, your patient will usually drop off when there is a perception of a lack of progress or when no more progress is being made. The step-by-step graded exposure programme combined with an effective explanation will solve this problem for the Go-To Therapist.

In the next chapter, we will dissect the essential components to ensuring you become the Go-To Therapist in your town, getting consistently long-lasting results and helping people who have failed traditional approaches and who travel miles to see you.

CHAPTER 18
A constraints-based physio approach – the fastest way to confidence and clarity

As you can hopefully see from the 12-step process outlined in the previous chapters, everything progresses logically in a systematic process.

The true secret, and some may say even hidden benefit, of the 12-step method is that it forces you to really focus your attention on getting the patient to the next step.

By keeping your attention laser-focused solely on getting the patient to the next step, something magical happens...

You don't get distracted treating the same area every session, magically hoping this week is the week the symptoms will settle down. And you don't throw a few exercises at the patient each session and, if they don't work, try a few different ones, until before you know it the patient has had five sessions and has got ten exercises to do three times a day...

...but rather you have one big goal per session and all your attention is focused on this. And with this laser focus, your attention is specifically on keeping that patient progressing. When the patient feels progress, can see the progress, and understands there is still more progress to be had, you will never have patients drop off, not show up or not adhere to your exercises.

Another big benefit of having a structured step-by-step system is that you will rarely need an hour for a session with a patient. A big myth is that therapists feel by giving patients longer, they are doing the patient a favour. The harsh truth is, the patient doesn't really care about the time: they care about the outcome.

To help you understand this, a good analogy I heard once in a business seminar is to imagine you are travelling on a seven-hour flight from

Manchester Airport to Boston, for example. The pilot comes on the public announcement service and says 'Great news – we've arrived at Boston one hour early and are hovering over Boston now for the next 60 minutes so you can get full value from your seven-hour flight.' You would be pretty angry with the pilot wouldn't you? You pay to get on the plane to get to the destination, not to waste an hour more than you need to.

This is the same in private practice. My aim with all our Go-To Therapists in my mentorship is to help them have the confidence and clarity to get even better results in just 30-minute sessions. If you are a therapist who gives your patients 60 minutes or even longer, 30 minutes might seem like a short space of time. The magical thing that confidence and clarity gives you is that you are actually working smarter, not harder, doing much less hands-on treatment, getting great changes in pain levels, range of motion and other KPIs and spending more time coaching the patient to be successful in key movements specific to their needs as part of the overall plan.

I actually find that 30 minutes is too long at times with the majority of patients now that I have a specific goal I need them to hit each session. If we progress through a couple of steps or progressions in the one session then, great, we simply find the limit of the patient's potential and hold them there with their movement plan until the next session as their nervous system adapts to the new load tolerance.

Obviously there will be a small minority of patients who will need longer than 30 minutes during some sessions, but for the majority of cases, you can make a lot of progress in a short space of time if you are working smarter not harder.

Working smarter not harder will save your hands, double your income for the same amount of hours worked and allow you to have laser focus in each session with every patient's movement plan bespoke to their needs. This will take away the 'boredom' and 'monotony' that so many therapists experience from saying the same things over and over again every single day, dishing out the same exercises regardless of the person's story and desired destination.

How much more income could you make in your practice by getting your sessions down to 30 minutes while getting better and more consistent results and making a meaningful impact to all your patients' lives?

Forget about limiting beliefs of pathology or past experiences, or how many therapists they have seen before you; treat every person as an individual and work smarter not harder. This constraints-based approach is the quickest way I know to ethically grow your business by improving your retention, referrals, revenue and reputation/recognition as the Go-To Therapist in your town by getting meaningful results that add so much value to your patients' lives.

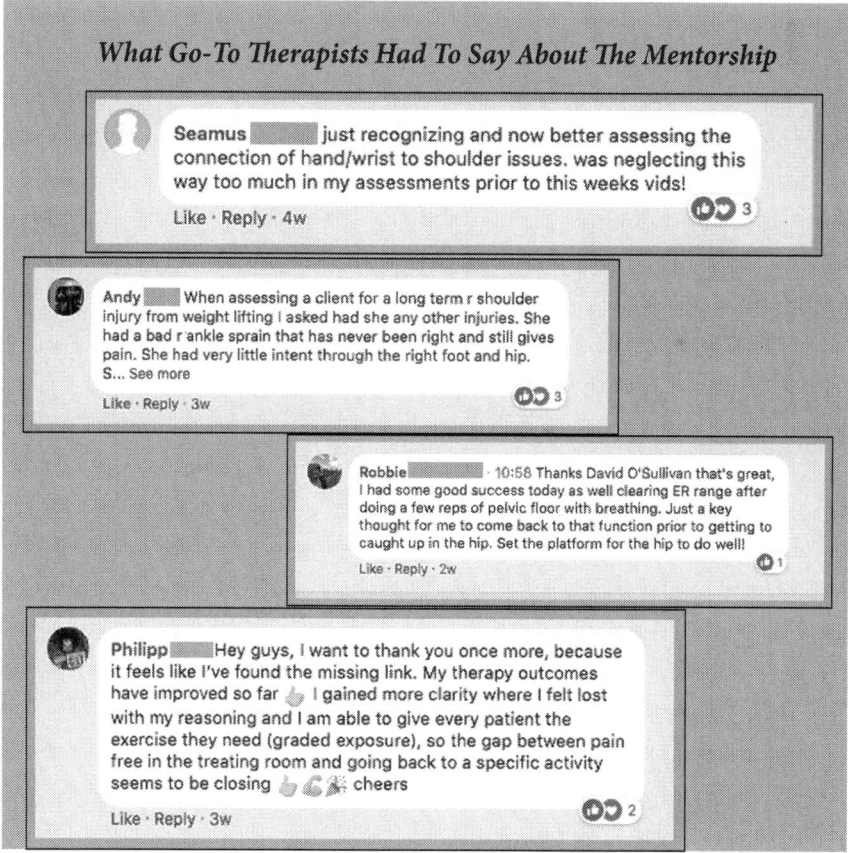

What Go-To Therapists Had To Say About The Mentorship

Seamus [ ] just recognizing and now better assessing the connection of hand/wrist to shoulder issues. was neglecting this way too much in my assessments prior to this weeks vids!

Like · Reply · 4w

Andy [ ] When assessing a client for a long term r shoulder injury from weight lifting I asked had she any other injuries. She had a bad r ankle sprain that has never been right and still gives pain. She had very little intent through the right foot and hip. S... See more

Like · Reply · 3w

Robbie [ ] · 10:58 Thanks David O'Sullivan that's great, I had some good success today as well clearing ER range after doing a few reps of pelvic floor with breathing. Just a key thought for me to come back to that function prior to getting to caught up in the hip. Set the platform for the hip to do well!

Like · Reply · 2w

Philipp [ ] Hey guys, I want to thank you once more, because it feels like I've found the missing link. My therapy outcomes have improved so far 👍 I gained more clarity where I felt lost with my reasoning and I am able to give every patient the exercise they need (graded exposure), so the gap between pain free in the treating room and going back to a specific activity seems to be closing 👍👏 cheers

Like · Reply · 3w

CHAPTER 19

Building the go-to clinic

Building a Go-To Therapist practice isn't difficult if built on a solid foundation of being able to get consistently great, long-lasting results.

The principles and strategies can be applied to a chartered physiotherapist, physical therapist, sports therapist, sports rehabilitation therapist or sports massage therapist's practice wherever you are in the world.

I hear so many therapists saying they want to have a Go-To Therapist practice but, in reality, aren't actually willing to put the work in to achieve this. I would bet my life savings that there were not many therapists hungrier or more dedicated than I was in wanting to become the Go-To Therapist in my area when I first qualified, or many who put in the hours and hours of learning, application, tweaking, testing and repeating this process in both private practice and pro sport as I did.

I was obsessed (and still am) in becoming the Go-To Therapist that can help people who have failed traditional approaches, and give value back to their lives. I used to get a massive kick out of helping pro athletes and celebrities. The reality now for me is that I get much more satisfaction and reward helping 'non-sporting' patients get back to the simple things in life like getting up and down off a chair, or lifting their grandkids without being out of breath, in pain or discomfort, through moving more efficiently.

Luckily for you, you don't even need to spend a fraction of the time I put into getting to where I am today if you want to truly become the Go-To Therapist in your area. You just need to have passion for your work, care about your patients and a genuine interest in making a meaningful impact on every patient you come in contact with.

How much would a full diary and a consistent word-of-mouth referral system TRULY be worth to you and your family? £50,000 a year? Or actually £100,000+ a year if you truly have the confidence and 'know-how' to progress a patient through a FULL treatment plan EVEN IF they have seen numerous therapists before you?

If your patient ethically needs six sessions but you don't know how to progress them or clearly and logically EFFECTIVELY EXPLAIN WHY they need these sessions…

…or they feel like they are not making progress and drop off after four sessions, how much is that REALLY costing you, your business and your family?

The two extra sessions the patient ethically needed and the two filled slots in your diary?

Or the extra six-plus RETENTION sessions that patient may need with a new problem in the future?

Or the extra six-plus REFERRAL sessions from the person that the patient WOULD have sent you if you had got MEANINGFUL RESULTS?

You see, I see most therapists complaining about not being busy enough or not seeing enough patients EVEN THOUGH they've spent hundreds and hundreds of pounds on Facebook, Google Adwords and other marketing events when the TRUE PROBLEM is they actually don't have the CLARITY to:

1. **Make sense of the patient's story and make sense of the objective assessment.**

2. **Effectively explain to the patient the true problem but also the solution and the plan to get them to the desired destination.**

3. **Effectively implement a progressive step-by-step plan that gets results in the real world and ensures it is tailored to the patient's actual needs (and not just following your favourite exercises for these symptoms that work well with some patients but not others).**

4. **Know how to integrate their hands-on treatment with their progressive rehab exercises.**

5. Know when to push the patient but also when to back off.

6. Most importantly, know when the patient is ready to return to, and be successful with, the activities that are meaningful to their life and situation, even under times of high stress.

Sure, you might be OK for one to two sessions and change someone's pain experience short term but what happens when the patient's progress stalls or, worse, the pain returns with a vengeance and that 'novel' hands-on stimulus isn't so novel anymore and isn't working like it was in the first few sessions?

Where to then?

That's where the real money is leaking out of your business, or will be leaking out of your future business!!

Right now you might be thinking...

What would it be like to have that complete step-by-step system in place right now, with all of these steps solved on a day-to-day basis that **GETS YOU INCREASED REVENUE, REFERRALS and RECOGNITION?**

But let's step back to reality for a moment, and address the elephant in the room: None of this is possible if you don't focus on the ability to get consistent, long-lasting **RESULTS** by:

- Developing a relationship with your patient that forms a connection
- Researching what you need to spend 80% of your time, energy and effort on, specific to the person's story
- Reassuring the person and their nervous system
- Re-exposing them to appropriate levels of loading so they can thrive in the real world
- Empowering them to build resilience to the inevitable stressful events that they will be exposed to in their lives.

I've successfully implemented this system with therapists in numerous professional sports clubs and private practices around the world, and I did it by using the **ProSport Academy Go-To Therapist Mentorship Method** that I have outlined above.

The ProSport Academy Go-To Therapist Mentorship Method is HOW you get the right information from your patient, put it to use in your treatment plan and progress them at the right time without overwhelming or second-guessing yourself.

Then, make sure they can tolerate the demands placed upon their body specific to their situation so you can discharge them knowing with confidence that they have done everything that's needed to be resilient to the real world; they will have complete trust in you and your process; they will **return to you without a second thought in the future with new injuries** and **refer their closest family and friends to you**.

When you implement it, you get **CONSISTENT RESULTS** that allows you to **BECOME the biggest name in your town**. It's the fastest way I know to stop playing small and massively increase the demand for your services and **become known as the Go-To therapist that gives you financial freedom and a stress-free lifestyle.**

What is the alternative?

Take everything I have taught you throughout this book and start asking yourself some higher level questions and I have no doubt you will enjoy success with cases that would have left you frustrated in the past.

After all, what is the alternative?

The current approach to healthcare is obviously not working. Even in professional sport with so much sports science technology, hamstring injuries continue to remain as high as ever, ACL injuries are happening, recurring injuries are happening time and time again.

It is time to stand up and ask some common-sense, logical questions.

Why is that knee joint being overloaded in the first place? Why is the nerve root becoming sensitised in the first place?

Why is that rotator cuff becoming painful and weak in the first place?

Why is the gluteus medius 'weak' in the first place?

The answer always lies in the person's story.

Having worked with hundreds of therapists from professional sport, national healthcare settings and private practice, I can tell you what separates the world class Go-To Therapists from the average is the speed of implementation.

These Go-To Therapists don't look for excuses of 'I just need to wait a few months for this to happen first before I can get started' or 'I just don't have time for this now' or 'I don't have enough revenue at the moment to implement the changes I need'.

If you are good at what you do, you'll never be out of work.

Take this opportunity now before someone else comes in and implements these methods before your eyes and becomes the Go-To Therapist in your town.

Your Opportunity To Work Personally With Dave

I would like to take a moment to say thank you for giving me your time and attention right up until the end of this book. It tells me you have the passion and desire to become the Go-To Therapist in your town by first and foremost getting consistently great, long-lasting results that have a meaningful impact on your patients' lives.

This is exactly the type of person that I love to work with, and because of that I am offering you an opportunity to continue to study with me personally.

1 Free Online Training

The Go-To Therapist Blueprint Video Case Study:

> *'How To Take A Groin Pain Patient Who Has Seen Numerous Other Therapists & Get A Successful Patient Outcome That Allows You To Rapidly Raise Your Retention, Rates, Revenues, Referrals, and Recognition In Your Physio Practice.'*

The Go-To Therapist Blueprint Case Study is a free and in-depth online training webinar that shows you step-by-step videos of how my system looks in the real world with patients.

This 90-minute webinar will show you step-by-step (including example videos of exercises with real patients to look at) how people just like you have moved away from traditional physical therapy strategies of looking at the site of pain and strengthening it, which get some good results, to using the Go-To Therapist style that allows you to get consistent long-lasting results.

You will see proof that everything you have just read in the pages of this book really does work and that it can help you get more retention, referrals, revenue and recognition for your clinic and your family. I will be hosting this free online training personally, and you will be able to submit your questions beforehand.

Here's what you will learn:

- Step by step, the exact assessment, treatment and rehab system that Go-To Therapist students have used to add £12,000+ to their private practices within 90 days by increasing their retention, referrals, revenue and reputation by getting real world results with even the most tricky back pain cases.

- How one Go-To Therapist student left a physiotherapy clinic and started up on her own and is now getting a consistent word of mouth referral stream while being told 'no one has ever looked at me like this before', using the Go-To Therapist method.

- The exact progressions one therapist used to double his patient numbers, knowing he had everything he needed to build a Go-To Therapy clinic.

- How another therapist in Scotland charges what he truly believes he is worth now and enjoys coming to work each day getting consistently great results.

- A way that a Therapist in Trinidad and Tobago now manages acute low back pain patients.

ACCESS THE FREE TRAINING HERE:

www.thegotophysiobook.com/webinar

Choose this option if you want to see precisely how this system is being used by others just like you to bring in more retention of past patients, more referrals without even asking for them and a consistent increase in revenue. It is genuine training (90 minutes), and at the end of the training you will be given an opportunity to enrol in the Go-To Therapist Mentorship Programme, a 12-week Master Class where you can work personally with me if you decide it is right for you.

2 Work with me in the 12-week Go-To Therapist Online Mentorship Programme

The Go-To Therapist Mentorship Programme is a 12-week programme designed to help you build a Go-To Therapist practice in the quickest time possible, even if you are a new grad and have started up your own private practice.

In my Go-To Therapist Mentorship I'll show you how to effortlessly get a patient highly motivated, and following every single progressive exercise you prescribe so you BOTH get the results you want using the exact same system I've used with thousands of professional athletes and my own private practice.

BUT you also get paid what you truly and ethically deserve and have the cannonball effect kick into your business of more RETENTION, REFERRALS, REVENUE and RECOGNITION with your REPUTATION as the Go-To Therapist cemented in your town.

How long are you going to continue treating patients knowing you could be giving a better service while also improving your caseload and massively growing your reputation and business?

This Online Go-To Therapist Mentorship Programme isn't about overtreating patients or bringing them for extra sessions when they don't need them but rather guiding them through a step-by-step progressive programme that allows them to build resilience for themselves while adding massive value to their lives.

When you can get consistent, long-lasting results that add value to peoples' lives, you'll never have to worry about having a roller coaster revenue each month, a quiet diary and patients cancelling or not showing up.

The Go-To Therapist Mentorship Programme helps you gain a sound, clinically reasoned step-by-step process to treat the person in front of them, looking at the body as a whole and bringing that person back to their ideal outcome successfully, be it returning to training or sport, or non-sporting patients returning to activities of daily living.

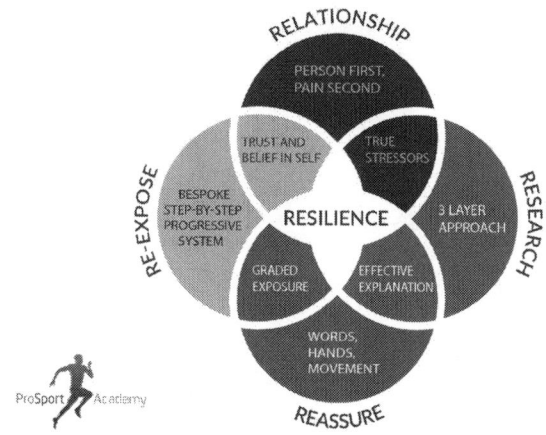

The online support and curriculum contains 12 modules (no longer than 1.5 hours per module) and the therapist has lifetime access to the content and the support of myself and my team.

This contains my EXACT assessments, explanations, treatment techniques, rehab exercises, protocols and high-end rehab and performance exercises that I use on a daily basis with world-class athletes but also with my private practice patients.

The Therapist Mentorship will show you how to assess a patient using a simple common-sense approach, how to find the true stressors that are causing the symptomatic tissues/muscle/joint to overload and how to design a systematic step-by-step progressive treatment plan for that person's specific needs.

You will then learn how to EFFECTIVELY EXPLAIN your findings and the plan that needs to happen so that the patient can get the ideal result they want.

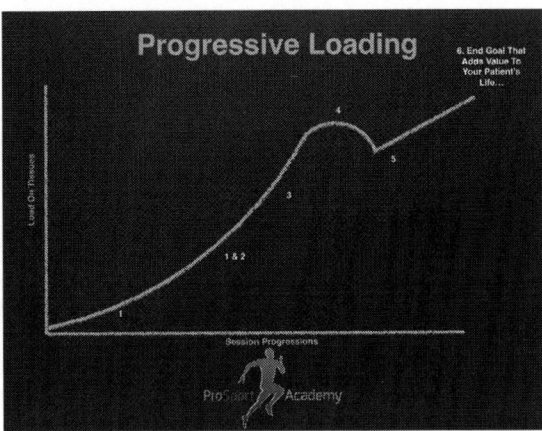

This ensures the patient completely understands the plan and how they will progress during every session, which eliminates drop-offs and patients not adhering to exercises or feeling like they are not making progress.

From here you will learn how to use hands-on treatment techniques (that are quick and effective and complement the rehab programme so your patient does not get reliant on just soft tissue treatment) and how to progress the loading of the tissues (that are not doing enough) using a systematic approach that I have used successfully in pro sport for the past ten years.

By the fourth session (sometimes longer depending on the presentation) you will actually be exposing your patient to GREATER loads in a safe manner in the clinic by your movement choice. They will need to be able to tolerate these in the real world with their first running session, for example.

When they can do these movements without any nervous system motor adaptations, you will logically prove to yourself that your patient is READY to go back to running or lifting weights or picking up their kids, or whatever goal your patient has.

You will know your patient is READY to get back to doing what they love without setbacks, flare-ups or recurrence of injuries and you constantly second-guessing yourself.

Give me 1% of your time for 12 weeks and I'll help you achieve more than you achieved in the last three years

Everything you need is delivered to you via a series of instant access videos, PDF 'cheat sheets', live Q/A calls (with me), and an interactive online community (of hundreds of other Go-To Therapist students), all to ensure that you can put this system into your practice without any hassle or getting stuck.

ACCESS THE GO-TO THERAPIST MENTORSHIP HERE:

www.thegotophysiobook.com/mentorship

If after reading this book you have decided that this type of method is exactly how you want to look at the body and get consistent real world results with your patients, and you do not want to wait another minute to have it working in your clinic, then go ahead and enroll in the programme now: **www.thegotophysiobook.com/enroll**

The best part is that most of my students see a return on their investment in the programme before they even finish it. My aim is to add AT LEAST £12,000 to your annual revenue within 90 days through getting consistently great results and having super fans as your patients.

So, what are you waiting for? Pick which one works best for you and let's get to work!

I'll see you on the webinar or in the advanced master class Go-To Therapist Mentorship Programme.

To your business success, your reputation and your patients' improved quality of life.

Dave O'Sullivan

P.S. If you are really done with just treating the symptoms and getting some OK results but some that won't respond; if you are done with patients not adhering to your exercises and losing motivation; if you are really committed to doing what it takes to achieve the consistent results you and your patients desire and deserve; if you are serious about achieving your full professional potential and becoming a successful profitable business owner – then I am committed to helping you achieve it.

I am the 'perfect' guide for you and I want you to know that everything I teach is what I use in the real world with my own professional athletes and private practice patients to get real world results.

I've spent thousands of hours and pounds learning everything that I've shared with you in this book. Investing in myself and my clinical and business education is the only reason that I am in a position to write a book like this as the present England Rugby League Physiotherapist. I was not the smartest in my class or scoring massive percentages in my essays in university. I paid to learn the path in the real world with a patient in front of me in my clinic. Every bit of it.

Investing in myself and my education with the right people is the sole reason I was able to achieve my dream job of working with Munster Rugby Union after only four years of graduating, as well as having the confidence to start a private practice from scratch in Huddersfield, one year after graduating, that's now allowed me to take care of my own and my family's long-term future while getting paid what I'm worth and delivering life-changing results to so many of my patients.

Despite having invested well over £200,000 in clinical and business education now, and consistently investing £20,000+ per year, I can tell you the greatest investment was investing in the right people who were two or three steps ahead of where I wanted to be.

A successful, profitable business is the EFFECT of my actions. Investing in myself was the CAUSE.

If you want the appropriate training (the CAUSE) to grow your results, reputation and business successfully (the EFFECT), please contact me through email with any questions you might have or take action via the opportunities listed below:

Email: **dave@thegotophysio.com**

To take the FREE webinar:

www.thegotophysiobook.com/webinar

To take the advanced Go-To Therapist Mentorship Masterclass Programme with me:

www.thegotophysiobook.com/mentorship

Aout Dave O'Sullivan

Dave O'Sullivan is the current England Rugby League Physiotherapist and private practice owner, originally from Cork, Ireland.

Dave is the founder of The ProSport Academy Ltd. – an online mentoring company he set up to help therapists become the Go-To Therapist in their area in 2015. Since 2015, Dave has worked with hundreds of professional sports physios, private practice therapists, strength coaches, rehab coaches and sports massage therapists with his method and systems helping people that have failed traditional approaches in clinics all over the world.

Dave also has grown ProSport Physiotherapy Huddersfield Ltd. – a successful private practice that helps both professional athletes and members of the general public get back to the things they love doing in life, pain-free from a one-room treatment room above a running shop to a five treatment room private practice with a yoga studio and 14 full-time staff. Dave has now helped the therapists working in his clinic become the Go-To Therapists in his own town of Huddersfield who make a meaningful impact on their patients' lives.

Dave is the host of the Go-To Physio show (available on Youtube, Itunes, Soundcloud and Stitcher). The Go-To Physio show helps therapists gain the confidence and clarity to get consistent, long-lasting results that allow them to rapidly increase their retention, referrals, revenue and recognition as the Go-To Therapist.

Dave is widely regarded as the Go-To Therapist in Rugby League and consults with numerous clubs and athletes. He also works with professional golfers, GAA players and athletes in numerous other sports.

Every week, thousands of therapists receive his support/advice online and attend his seminars. His Go-To Therapist Mentorship has sold out the past three times it has opened for enrollment.

Key reference papers that have influenced my thought process

Blackburn JT, Padua DA. Influence of trunk flexion on hip and knee joint kinematics during a controlled drop landing. *Clin Biomech* (Bristol, Avon). 2008; 23 (3): 313–9.

Bosch, F. and Van Hooren, B . (2016). Influence of Muscle Slack on High-Intensity Sport Performance: A Review. *Strength And Conditioning Journal*. 38 (5), p75–87.

Chaudhry H, Schleip R, Ji Z, Bukiet B, Maney M, Findley T. Three-dimensional mathematical model for deformation of human fasciae in manual therapy. *J Am Osteopath Assoc*. 2008; 108 (8): 379–90.

Courtney, R. (2009). The functions of breathing and its dysfunctions and their relationship to breathing therapy. *International Journal of Osteopathic Medicine*. 12 (3), p78–85.

Dyhre-poulsen P, Krogsgaard MR. Muscular reflexes elicited by electrical stimulation of the anterior cruciate ligament in humans. *J Appl Physiol*. 2000; 89 (6): 2191–5.

Farina D, Arendt-nielsen L, Graven-nielsen T. Experimental muscle pain reduces initial motor unit discharge rates during sustained submaximal contractions. *J Appl Physiol*. 2005; 98 (3): 999–1005.

Fukui T, Otake Y, Kondo T. In which direction does skin move during joint movement?. *Skin Res Technol*. 2016; 22 (2): 181–8.

Gregory JE, Wise AK, Wood SA, Prochazka A, Proske U. Muscle history, fusimotor activity and the human stretch reflex. *J Physiol* (Lond). 1998; 513 (Pt 3): 927–34.

Harper CJ, Shahgholi L, Cieslak K, Hellyer NJ, Strommen JA, Boon AJ. Variability in diaphragm motion during normal breathing, assessed with B-mode ultrasound. *J Orthop Sports Phys Ther.* 2013; 43 (12): 927–31.

Hodges PW, Coppieters MW, Macdonald D, Cholewicki J. New insight into motor adaptation to pain revealed by a combination of modelling and empirical approaches. *Eur J Pain.* 2013; 17 (8): 1138–46.

Hodges PW, Ervilha UF, Graven-nielsen T. Changes in motor unit firing rate in synergist muscles cannot explain the maintenance of force during constant force painful contractions. *J Pain.* 2008; 9 (12): 1169–74.

Hodges PW, Smeets RJ. Interaction between pain, movement, and physical activity: short-term benefits, long-term consequences, and targets for treatment. *Clin J Pain.* 2015; 31 (2): 97–107.

Hug F, Hodges PW, Carroll TJ, De martino E, Magnard J, Tucker K. Motor Adaptations to Pain during a Bilateral Plantarflexion Task: Does the Cost of Using the Non-Painful Limb Matter?. *PLoS ONE.* 2016; 11 (4): e0154524.

Hug F, Hodges PW, Tucker K. Task dependency of motor adaptations to an acute noxious stimulation. *J Neurophysiol.* 2014; 111 (11): 2298–306.

Johansson H, Sjölander P, Sojka P. Receptors in the knee joint ligaments and their role in the biomechanics of the joint. *Crit Rev Biomed Eng.* 1991; 18 (5): 341–68.

Maas H, Baan GC, Huijing PA. Muscle force is determined also by muscle relative position: isolated effects. *J Biomech.* 2004; 37 (1): 99–110.

Mason-mackay AR, Whatman C, Reid D. The effect of reduced ankle dorsiflexion on lower extremity mechanics during landing: A systematic review. *J Sci Med Sport.* 2017; 20 (5): 451–458.

Morin JB, Gimenez P, Edouard P, et al. Sprint Acceleration Mechanics: The Major Role of Hamstrings in Horizontal Force Production. *Front Physiol.* 2015; 6: 404.

Moritz CT, Farley CT. Passive dynamics change leg mechanics for an unexpected surface during human hopping. *J Appl Physiol.* 2004; 97 (4): 1313–22.

Moseley GL, Hodges PW. Reduced variability of postural strategy prevents normalization of motor changes induced by back pain: a risk factor for chronic trouble?. *Behav Neurosci.* 2006; 120 (2): 474–6.

Prior S, Mitchell T, Whiteley R, et al. The influence of changes in trunk and pelvic posture during single leg standing on hip and thigh muscle activation in a pain free population. *BMC Sports Sci Med Rehabil.* 2014; 6 (1): 13.

Roeder BA, Kokini K, Sturgis JE, Robinson JP, Voytik-harbin SL. Tensile mechanical properties of three-dimensional type I collagen extracellular matrices with varied microstructure. *J Biomech Eng.* 2002; 124 (2): 214–22.

Scarfe AC, Li FX, Reddin DB, Bridge MW. A new progression scale for common lower-limb rehabilitation tasks. *J Strength Cond Res.* 2011; 25 (3): 612–9.

Schleip R, Naylor IL, Ursu D, et al. Passive muscle stiffness may be influenced by active contractility of intramuscular connective tissue. *Med Hypotheses.* 2006; 66 (1): 66–71.

Shacklock MO. Central pain mechanisms: A new horizon in manual therapy. *Aust J Physiother.* 1999; 45 (2): 83–92.

Sokoloff AJ, Siegel SG, Cope TC. Recruitment order among motoneurons from different motor nuclei. *J Neurophysiol.* 1999; 81 (5): 2485–92.

Solomonow M. Ligaments: a source of work-related musculoskeletal disorders. *J Electromyogr Kinesiol.* 2004;14(1):49-60.

Tanaka H, Ikezoe T, Umehara J, et al. Influences of Fascicle Length During Isometric Training on Improvement of Muscle Strength. *J Strength Cond Res.* 2016; 30 (11): 3249–3255.

Teng HL, Powers CM. Hip-Extensor Strength, Trunk Posture, and Use of the Knee-Extensor Muscles During Running. *J Athl Train.* 2016; 51 (7): 519–24.

Teng HL, Powers CM. Influence of trunk posture on lower extremity energetics during running. *Med Sci Sports Exerc.* 2015; 47 (3): 625–30.

Teyhen DS, Shaffer SW, Butler RJ, et al. What Risk Factors Are Associated With Musculoskeletal Injury in US Army Rangers? A Prospective Prognostic Study. *Clin Orthop Relat Res.* 2015; 473 (9): 2948–58.

Thacker, M. (2015). Louis Gifford – Revolutionary: The Mature Organism Model, an embodied cognitive perspective of pain. *In Touch.* 152 (1), p4–9.

Tucker KJ, Hodges PW. Changes in motor unit recruitment strategy during pain alters force direction. *Eur J Pain.* 2010; 14 (9): 932–8.

Tucker KJ, Hodges PW, Van den hoorn W, Nordez A, Hug F. Does stress within a muscle change in response to an acute noxious stimulus?. *PLoS ONE.* 2014; 9 (3): e91899.

Van der krogt MM, De graaf WW, Farley CT, Moritz CT, Richard casius LJ, Bobbert MF. Robust passive dynamics of the musculoskeletal system compensate for unexpected surface changes during human hopping. *J Appl Physiol.* 2009; 107 (3): 801–8.

Verkuil B, Brosschot JF, Tollenaar MS, Lane RD, Thayer JF. Prolonged Non-metabolic Heart Rate Variability Reduction as a Physiological Marker of Psychological Stress in Daily Life. *Ann Behav Med.* 2016; 50 (5): 704–714.

Index

Printed in Great Britain
by Amazon